ATKINS DIET

Easier to Follow than Keto, Paleo, Mediterranean or Low-Calorie Diet, Allows You to Lose Weight Quickly, Without Saying Goodbye to Sweets & Ice Cream Super Prohibited & Desired in a Diet!

BY

Jessica Davidson

Table Of Contents

Introduction

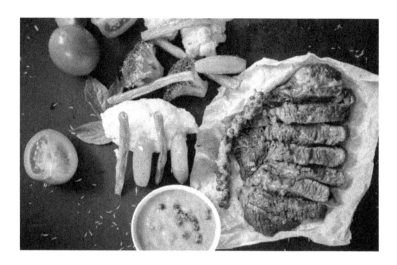

An Introduction to ATKINS Diet

What is Atkins Diet?

The Atkins Diet was created by Dr. Robert Atkins, a cardiologist whose interest in the health benefits of low-carb diets first culminated in the 1972 book "Dr. Atkins Diet Revolution," The diet involves four phases, starting with very few carbs and eating progressively more until you get to your desired weight. In phase one, for example, you're allowed 20 grams a day of "net carbs," 12 to 15 of them from "foundation vegetables" high in fiber like arugula, cherry tomatoes and Brussels sprouts, according to the traditional Atkins 20 plan. This is advised for maximum weight loss. Two other iterations of the diet, Atkins 40, which the company says is "perfect for those who have less than 40 pounds to lose," and Atkins 100, a plan promoted to those seeking to maintaining their current weight, have a starting point of 40 grams and 100 grams of net carbs per day, respectively.

Generally speaking, the theory is that by limiting carbs, your body has to turn to an alternative fuel – stored fat. So sugars and "simple starches" like potatoes, white bread and rice are all but squeezed out; protein and fat like chicken, meat and eggs are embraced. Fat is burned; pounds come off.

But reducing total carbs isn't all there is to Atkins. Limiting the carbs you take in at any one time is also in the game plan. A carb-heavy meal floods the blood with glucose, too much for the cells to use or to store in the liver as glycogen. Where does it end up? As fat.

In terms of plan flexibility, Atkins 100 allows you to eat the widest variety of foods in the beginning, allocating 100 net carbs throughout the day. Here's how it breaks down:

- A minimum of 12 to 15 grams of net carbs a day of foundation vegetables
- Three 4- to 6-ounce servings of protein a day
- Two to four servings of added fat a day

The remaining 85 grams of net carbs come from foods like legumes, nuts or seeds, higher-carb fruits and vegetables and whole grains.

Low-Carb Diet

These diets provide fewer carbs than is recommended by government guidelines and are known to bring on quick weight loss.

How much does Atkins Diet cost?

Meat and fresh veggies are pricier than most processed and fast foods, so the Atkins Diet is typically more expensive than the average American's. How much more than usual you'll spend will depend largely on your choices of protein sources. Are you buying mostly ground beef or springing for veal? Chicken or turkey? Chuck vs. New York strip? Buying in season should keep the veggie tab reasonable.

Will Atkins Diet help you lose weight?

Atkins and other low-carb diets have been studied longer and harder than most other approaches, and Atkins does appear to be moderately successful, especially in the first couple of weeks. That's only part of the story, however.

Much of the initial loss is water, say experts, because of the diet's diuretic effect. That's true of many other diets, too, and is one of the reasons researchers don't judge diets based on a few weeks of results. In diet studies, long-term generally starts at two years. Here's what several key studies had to say about Atkins and other low-carb diets:

Over short periods, Atkins results vary. In one study, published in 2006 in the British Medical Journal, Atkins dieters lost an average of 10 pounds in the first four weeks while those on meal-replacement (Slim Fast), caloric-restriction (Weight Watchers) and low-fat (Rosemary Conley's "Eat Yourself Slim" book) diets lost 6 to 7 pounds. At the one-month point and thereafter, however, there were no significant differences in weight loss among the groups.

A 2007 study that appeared in the Journal of the American Medical Association divided roughly 300 overweight or obese women into groups and assigned them to one of four types of diets: low-carb (Atkins), low-fat (Ornish), low saturated-fat/moderate-carb (LEARN), and roughly equal parts protein, fat, and carb (Zone). At two months, the Atkins dieters had lost an average of about 9½ pounds compared with 5 to 6 pounds for those on the other three diets. At six months, weight loss for the Atkins group averaged about 13 pounds; the other three groups averaged 4 1/2 to 7 pounds. At 12 months, the Atkins group had lost what researchers called a "modest" 10 pounds; the other dieters averaged 3 1/2 to 6 pounds. Drawing firm conclusions from this study is risky, however. The dropout rate in all four groups was significant, and many participants didn't follow their assigned diet. The Atkins dieters, for example, took in far more carbs than they were supposed to.

A third study, published in 2010 in the Annals of Internal Medicine, found no clear advantage either to a low-carb diet based on Atkins or a generic low-fat diet. Both helped participants lose an average of 11% of their starting weight at 12 months, but they gained about a third of it back after that. At two years, average loss for both diets was 7% of initial body weight. (That's still not bad – if you're overweight, losing just 5 to 10% of your current weight can help stave off some diseases.) An analysis of five studies that compared low-carb and low-fat diets published in 2006 in the Archives of Internal Medicine concluded similarly – while weight loss was greater at six months for low-carb dieters, by 12 months that difference wasn't significant.

It is still unclear, regardless of claims made for low-carb diets, whether the main reason for weight loss is carb restriction specifically or simply cutting calories. A study published in 2009 in the New England Journal of Medicine found that after two years, participants assigned either to a 35% or a 65% carb diet lost about the same amount of weight – 6 to 7 1/2 pounds on average. In 2003, researchers who analyzed about 100 low-carb studies concluded in the Journal of the American Medical Association that weight loss on those diets was associated mostly with cutting calories and not with cutting carbs.

Researchers reviewed 17 different studies that followed a total of 1,141 obese patients on low-carb eating plans, some similar to the Atkins diet. Results were published in 2012 in Obesity. The study shows that low-carb dieters lost an average of nearly 18 pounds over a period of six months to a year. They also saw improvements in their waist circumference.

In a study published in November 2014 in Circulation: Cardiovascular Quality and Outcomes, researchers analyzed existing research on Atkins, South Beach, Weight Watchers and the Zone diets to find out which was most effective. Their findings suggested that none of the four diet plans led to significant weight loss, and none was starkly better than the others when it came to keeping weight off for a year or more. Each of the four plans helped dieters shed about the same number of pounds in the short term: around 5% of their starting body weight. After two years, however, some of the lost weight was regained by those on the Atkins or Weight Watchers plans. Since the diets produce similar results, the study authors concluded that dieters should choose the one that best adheres to their lifestyle – for example, Weight Watchers involved a group-based, behavior-modification approach, and Atkins focuses on lowering carbs.

Following the Atkins Diet will likely seriously challenge your willpower. How much do you love sweet and starchy foods? Would you miss crusty French bread? Pasta? Grape jelly? Diets that severely limit entire food groups for months and years tend to have lower success rates than less-restrictive diets do, and the Atkins Diet is the definition of a restrictive diet.

One study showed higher percentages of Atkins dieters dropping out at three, six, 12 and 24 months than others did on a low-fat diet, but the differences were not significant. Two other studies that included low-carb dieters concluded diet type wasn't connected to dropout rate.

The Atkins Diet isn't known for its convenience. At home, building variety into meals is a little harder than usual. Eating out takes more effort. Alcohol is limited. Company products and online resources may be helpful. In 2013, Atkins launched a frozen-food line, which the company says is the first low-carb frozen-food line on the market.

Atkins recipes abound. Atkins provides meal plans, recipes with ingredient lists and food carb counts, all in print-friendly format. There is at least a smattering of recipes across a range of cuisines from American to Middle Eastern to French to Asian.

Eating out is doable on the Atkins Diet. Just make sure you've read Atkins' list of approved fast-food and cuisine-specific options before heading out (and don't be bashful about asking lots of questions about meal preparation).

Chapter 1:
How Does Atkins Diet Works?

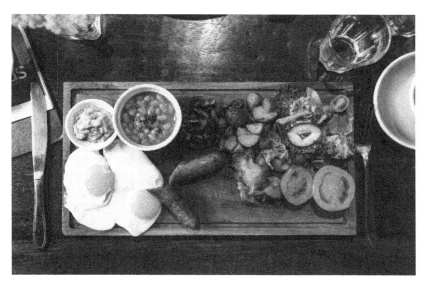

How It Works

The Atkins diet plan relies on knowing how much carbohydrate is in everything you eat. Specifically, consumers count their net carbs. Net carbs can be calculated by checking the total grams of carbohydrate in your portion of food and subtracting the grams of fiber and sugar alcohols or glycerin (if applicable).

There are three Atkins programs based on different levels of net carb intake per day. The company recommends that you check with your healthcare provider for personalized advice before choosing a program to manage a medical condition.

Atkins 20

The Atkins 20 plan is what most would consider to be the classic Atkins plan. It is designed for those who have over 40 pounds to lose, have a waist size of over 35 (for women) or 40 (for men), are pre-diabetic, or diabetic. People on this program start by consuming just 20 net carbs per day. They eat a variety of approved (foundational) vegetables, lean meat, cheese, and healthy fats to meet their energy needs. After two weeks on Atkins 20, people on this plan can begin to add berries, nuts, and other fiber-rich carb sources in five net carb increments. Then gradually they learn to incorporate healthier carbohydrate choices to reach and maintain their goal weight.

There are four phases to the Atkins 20 program:

Induction Phase. For two weeks or longer, consumers keep their net carbs at the lowest level.

Balancing Phase. People on the program slowly add grams of net carbs to find the best carbohydrate balance.

Fine Tuning Phase. Clients are advised make small tweaks to reach and maintain their goal weight for at least a month.

Lifetime Maintenance. You continue to eat a healthy diet with limited carbohydrates to maintain your goal weight.

Atkins 40

This plan offers a more relaxed program where dieters eat from all food groups from day one. The plan is designed for people who have 40 pounds or less to lose, those who prefer a wider variety of food choices, or for women who are breastfeeding with a goal to lose weight. On this program, you start the first phase of the plan by consuming 40 grams of net carbs per day from vegetables, fruits, nuts, legumes, and whole grains. As dieters approach their goal weight, they add carbs in 10 net carb increments to find their personal carb "sweet spot" to maintain their healthy weight.

Atkins 100

This is the most relaxed Atkins eating program. It is designed for those who want to maintain their current weight, who prefer the widest variety of food choices, or for women who are breastfeeding and have a goal to maintain weight. The company also suggests this program for women who are pregnant as long as they have approval from their healthcare provider. On this plan, you consume about 100 grams of net carb per day with no foods that are off limits.

On each of the Atkins plans, net carbs are to be divided between three meals and two snacks per day so that blood sugar remains stable throughout the day. You don't count calories on these programs, but portion size recommendations are provided. Additionally, it recommended that certain foods (such as added fats) are limited.

Pros and Cons

Consumers who choose to go on an Atkins eating plan are likely to see some weight loss and health benefits.

For many people, restricting carbohydrates means eliminating heavily processed, high-sugar, high-starch foods which contribute calories without substantial nutrition.

If you replace those less healthy foods with more nutritious foods (such as those on the Atkins Acceptable Foods lists), you are likely to increase your intake of important micro and macronutrients.

On the flip side, however, if you currently consume a standard American diet, adjusting to an Atkins plan may be challenging, especially if you choose to go on the Atkins 20 plan. Typically, people consume most of their calories from carbohydrate. Cutting back on carbs can lead to symptoms including headaches, fatigue, mood swings, and constipation.

Additionally, even though you don't have to count calories on the Atkins diet, you do need to count carbs, calculate net carbs and balance carbs between meals and snacks. You'll also need to use food lists to make sure you're consuming foods that are compliant. For many busy people, this work may seem overwhelming. As an alternative, consumers can choose to purchase an Atkins meal plan and get pre-packaged meals, smoothies, and snacks.

Pros

If you are interested in the Atkins diet, there are substantial studies documenting the benefits of going on the low-carb diet. Many of these published studies have supported the use of the program for weight loss and other health benefits.

Weight Loss

The Atkins diet has a long history of successful weight loss. Many people have lost weight on this plan and the program has been studied in numerous clinical trials. But if you are considering Atkins for weight loss or weight maintenance, you'll find that there is a range of studies with conflicting results.

A study published in JAMA compared the Atkins diet to LEARN (Lifestyle, Exercise, Attitudes, Relationships, and Nutrition, a program that is low in fat and high in carbohydrate based on national guidelines), Zone, and Ornish diets in overweight pre-menopausal women. Researchers found that those following Atkins lost more weight and experienced more favorable overall metabolic effects at 12 months.

Another analysis of studies published in the journal Nutrients compared Atkins to 19 other diets without specific calories targets. The researchers determined that of the diets evaluated, the Atkins diet showed the most evidence in producing clinically meaningful short-term and long-term weight loss.

However, there is also substantial research comparing high fat ketogenic diets (such as Atkins) to diets where calories are restricted. Several of these studies have shown that there is no difference between caloric restriction and carb restriction for long-term weight loss. Additionally, while there is some support for low-carb, higher fat diets, there are still medical experts who question whether or not the diet is healthy or effective for the long-term.

Results from a large nutritional study were reported in 2019 at both the American Society of Nutrition and the American Diabetes Association conferences. The findings suggest that there isn't necessarily a single diet that meets the needs of every person trying to lose weight because each body responds differently. These findings support research published in other scientific journals suggesting that the best diet for weight loss is the diet you can stick to for the long-term.

Some studies have demonstrated that Atkins and other ketogenic diets are effective for weight loss. However, other studies have concluded that cutting carbs is no more effective than cutting calories, especially over the long-term. This has led many researchers to suggest that the best eating and lifestyle program for weight loss and weight maintenance is the plan you can stick to for life.

No Calorie Counting

There is growing frustration over the use of calorie counting for weight loss and weight maintenance. Even though most nutrition experts acknowledge the importance of consuming the right number of calories each day, they acknowledge that trying to track and monitor your intake every day can be tedious and may feel restrictive.

On the Atkins plan, you watch your net carb intake but there is no need to count or restrict calories. For many people, this feature of the Atkins plan is most appealing.

Hearty Eating Plan

Some people like the fact that you can eat more rich and satisfying food on the Atkins diet plan. For example, some people prefer this diet because hearty foods like steaks and burgers can stay on their menu.

Protein-rich foods and foods with more fat tend to be satiating. When you feel satisfied after eating, you're likely to delay your next meal or snack and may consume fewer calories overall as a result. In fact, some studies have shown that total caloric intake is lower on the Atkins plan than on other plans with higher carbohydrate intake. It is important to note, however, that the most current versions of Atkins provide recommendations for portion size. For example, during Phase 1, the recommended daily intake for added fat is just 2–4 tablespoons. So you can't expect to be successful on the Atkins plan if you eat large portions of fatty meat, butter, and cheese.

Clearly Defined Guidelines

Those who prefer a structured approach to eating will enjoy Atkins. Each phase of the program has a specific time or weight goal that is clearly explained. For example, Phase 1 lasts for two weeks (in most situations). Phase 2 lasts until you are 10 pounds from your goal weight. Phase 3 lasts until have been comfortably at your goal weight for four weeks. Extensive lists of acceptable foods are available for each stage and portion sizes for each food category are clearly defined.

Focus on Healthy Carbs

The Atkins diet eliminates refined carbohydrates such as baked goods (like cake and white bread) and encourages the intake of healthy carbohydrates (such as green vegetables and fiber-rich berries), especially in the later stages of the plan. So you learn the difference between good carbs and bad carbs.

For many people, simply reducing the intake of refined grains and sugary foods provides noticeable benefits right away. Drinking water instead of soda and replacing starchy side dishes with foundation vegetables is likely to help you have steady energy levels throughout the day. In addition, you'll lose water weight almost immediately if you cut back on your carb intake.

Resources Widely Available

You'll find most of what you need to follow the Atkins plan online. Food lists and other guides are provided on their website. You'll also find Atkins books and guides in bookstores and online. If you don't like to prepare your own food all the time, Atkins snack bars and other meal replacements are conveniently available in many markets and discount stores.

Cons

While some dieters enjoy the diet's benefits, others struggle to stick to Atkins' strict eating plan.

Reduced Fruit and Grain Intake

If you're a person who loves fruit, you might struggle on the Atkins plan. Even if you don't love fruit, the USDA recommends that you consume about two cups per day to get the important vitamins and nutrients that they provide.

Eventually, you can add some fruit but in the early stages of the diet, you'll need to avoid healthy foods like berries, bananas, apple, and citrus fruits in order to get into ketosis. Once you are closer to your goal weight, you may be able to consume small amounts of low-carb fruits (such as raspberries) but some people aren't able to stay in ketosis when they consume any fruit. Grain intake is another concern on the Atkins diet. On the Atkins diet grain-based foods are restricted—especially in the early phases.

Chapter 2:
The Benefits Of The Atkins Diet

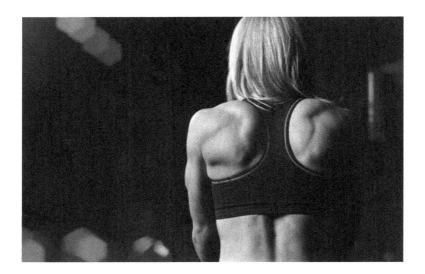

15 Health Benefits of the Atkins Diet

What are the health benefits of the Atkins diet?

This diet is usually recommended for people who are looking for a fairly quick way to achieve weight loss goals, but eating a low-carb diet will provide individuals with a wide range of valuable health benefits.

There have been more than 20 different studies to look at how this diet impacts weight loss and leads to other health improvements, and the diet has become a popular option around the world for people seeking enhanced wellness – without the stress of constantly monitoring your calorie intake.

One: The Atkins diet will improve your heart health.

Researchers who examined 17 different studies of overweight people found that following a low-carb, high-fat diet had a 98 per cent greater chance of lowering the risk of stroke or heart attack than a low-fat diet. Because of how carbohydrates trigger your body to rapidly produce insulin, you'll also end up holding onto excess fat for your body to use as fuel later, when your blood sugar crashes.

Cutting your intake of carbohydrates had a direct impact on your heart health several ways – decreasing your level of triglycerides, raising your levels of "good" cholesterol's, lowering your "bad" cholesterols, and even helping to reduce blood pressure.

Two: The Atkins diet will help you lose weight.

Some followers of the Atkins diet have managed to lose more than 100 pounds – but your individual weight loss results will depend heavily on your adherence to the plan. Since a low-carb diet helps stimulate your body to burn fat, and a diet high in protein and fat helps suppress your appetite, it's easy to see how the Atkins diet can lead to significant weight loss. However, you will need to pay close attention to the carbohydrate counts in everything you eat, as it can add up quickly and impede your potential weight loss results.

You'll see even better results if you mix in a bit of exercise. With the additional energy you'll have from eating clean and enjoying a strong metabolism, shoot for about 150 minutes each week of moderate-intensity exercise.

Three: The Atkins diet will improve blood sugar levels.

Uncontrolled sugar levels are a major risk factor for both heart disease and obesity – and the Atkins diet, particularly during the induction phase, can drastically improve your body's ability to properly process sugar. Even patients taking insulin before embarking on an Atkins diet were able to stop using insulin after changing their nutritional approach.

Limiting your intake of carbohydrates also helps to prevent blood sugar spikes, which are generally triggered by the glycemic content of high-carbohydrate foods. A low-glycemic diet is an effective way of dealing with that, but a low-glycemic diet combined with a reduced intake of carbohydrates is even better.

Four: The Atkins diet can prevent metabolic syndrome.

Most of the symptoms and risk factors that combine into what we know as metabolic syndrome can be treated with the nutritional approach of the Atkins diet. Abdominal obesity, elevated cholesterol, diabetes, and hypertension can all be addressed through this dietary strategy, and thanks to the healthy intake of protein, you can ensure that your muscle mass is preserved.

Maintaining muscle mass helps you keep your body's metabolism running efficiently, allowing you to continue burning fat and improving your overall wellness.

Five: The Atkins diet can help control your appetite.

You'll probably suffer through some cravings at first, especially during the induction phase as you try to cut out carbs almost entirely – but by eliminating the constant spikes and drops in your blood sugar, you'll enjoy a suppressed appetite. Not only will your Atkins diet help eliminate your cravings, you'll also be eating healthier meals more frequently, keeping you well-satiated.

If you do find yourself struggling with cravings, break up your meals with healthy snacks, drink more water, and make sure there isn't an emotional reason behind your physical food cravings. Once you get more familiar with your body, you'll be able to tell what's triggering your cravings and deal with them appropriately.

Six: The Atkins diet will boost brain function.

Low-carb diets have a reputation for negatively affecting your brain function, since your brain needs carbs for energy. However, once followers have gotten past the initial phase of reducing carbohydrate intake and their bodies have had a chance to adjust to a new metabolic process, the increased consumption of brain-healthy fats and B-complex vitamins found in leafy green vegetables work to produce more brain hormones like serotonin.

Low-carb fruits like berries also help enhance communication networks between your brain cells, promoting brain cell survival and regeneration.

Seven: The Atkins diet can provide increased physical endurance.

While scientists have long known how the Atkins diet can increase weight loss and the body's ability to effectively and efficiently burn fat, studies are now being done to examine how the diet could augment the body's physical performance and recovery.

According to some research, these athletes proved to be "very healthy," even "beyond what you can achieve with good genetics and extensive training," said Jeff Volek, lead researcher and professor of human sciences at the Ohio State University. Volek added that the restriction of carbs allows the body's fat-burning program to "reboot" and enable athletes to reach significantly improved levels of performance and health.

Eight: The Atkins diet can help clear your skin.

Studies have shown that the Atkins diet has a positive effect on a variety of chronic and unpleasant skin conditions – clearing up some of the redness, itching, and irritation associated with psoriasis, eczema, acne, and even vitiligo. Not only that, but even in practitioners without ongoing skin concerns, eating a low-carb diet can make your skin feel and look more radiant, moisturized, and healthy.

These benefits also impact your hair and your nails, which will all be stronger and healthier. The increased intake of vitamins and minerals you'll get from eating more vegetables and fruits will have a major effect how you feel inside and outside.

Nine: The Atkins diet will help you eat more nutrients.

By focusing your diet on whole, unprocessed foods, you'll enjoy eating far greater quantities of nutrients like vitamins, minerals, and antioxidants – all of which will directly impact your health and well-being. These nutrient-dense foods have a number of varied properties that will all provide a range of health benefits, which you wouldn't get if you were eating a plate of spaghetti or a pizza instead. Your meals should include an adequate portion of protein along with an array of high-fiber, low-glycemic fruits and vegetables. This encourages you to eat different kinds of produce and get different kinds of nutrients, achieving a well-balanced, healthy diet.

Ten: The Atkins diet will decrease inflammation.

Inflammation is an important part of your body's defense system, and a certain amount is to be expected in any healthy individual – especially during times of illness or injury. However, chronic inflammation can lead to serious health concerns like cancer, heart disease, and even neurological disorders like Alzheimer's and Parkinson's.

A lot of this inflammation can be attributed to the insulin spikes that come from eating processed foods and sugars, including carbs. Eating a variety of foods that decrease inflammation, like those recommended on the Atkins diet, can prevent chronic inflammation from causing lasting damage.

Eleven: The Atkins diet will improve digestion.

While your digestive system will likely need a bit of time to adjust to your new eating habits, a low-carb diet has proven to improve overall digestion. Thanks to the increased fiber intake found within the Atkins diet, you'll enjoy a heathy digestive system and reduced acid reflux, heartburn, and bloating.

Initially, you may find you are more flatulent than usual, but as your body gets used to your nutritional intake, you'll find that you suffer from gas less, as well.

Twelve: The Atkins diet can help prevent cancer.

A nutrition plan that focuses on getting enough healthy fats can drastically reduce your chances of developing certain types of cancers. Cancer growth happens when your body is running inefficiently, creating a breeding ground for developing infections. Uncontrolled blood sugar is a major trigger for this development, but the Atkins diet has proven effective at keeping these levels stable. The reduced inflammation also helps keep your body's immune response functioning effectively, and helps your body react effectively to stress.

Thirteen: The Atkins diet targets abdominal fat deposits.

Excess fat that has accumulated around your midsection can lead to a number of health risks – impacting almost every organ in your body by producing excess chemicals and hormones.

Major concerns include type 2 diabetes, colorectal cancer, and cardiovascular disease.

This fat is troublesome to lose and easy to put on, but can be reduced thanks to three major factors – exercise, sleep, and diet. The Atkins diet gives you the tools to tackle all three, starting with your nutritional intake.

Fourteen: The Atkins diet can enhance sleep quality.

With your increased consumption of nutrients, healthy amounts of fat and protein, and stable blood sugar, your body will be under less stress and feeling much healthier and more energetic. This will dramatically reduce the time you spend fighting insomnia, meaning you'll be able to fall asleep faster and stay asleep longer.

The quality of your rest will also be improved thanks to the brain-boosting power of the Atkins diet, and the added energy you'll see from all the nutrients you're putting in your body.

Fifteen: The Atkins diet helps with weight maintenance.

Once you've reached the fourth phase of the Atkins diet, you'll be in maintenance mode. With most diets, followers use this as an opportunity to return to their regular eating habits – and will end up piling all that lost weight right back on.

However, since Atkins is considered a life-long nutritional approach instead of a temporary diet, you'll have much better luck maintaining your weight loss and health benefits. Introduce carbohydrates slowly, and if you start having cravings, lower your intake. Switching between the third and fourth phases while keeping an eye on your overall health is a great way to keep those pounds off and enjoy the healthy lifestyle Atkins delivers.

What should I keep in mind when starting this diet?

If these great health benefits have convinced you to cut down on your carbohydrate intake and begin eating an Atkins-inspired diet, there are some things you should keep in mind as you set out on your new journey. While the benefits of the Atkins diet far outweigh any of the challenges that come along with it, it's important to know what obstacles you might come across – especially during your first few weeks on the diet.

Fortunately, you'll feel so good on this diet that you'll have no trouble overlooking these minor issues. It's easy to make a change when you know how huge the payoff is – and the Atkins diet is a great step along the way to lasting health and wellness.

Carb crash is a real thing.

When you're used to eating plenty of carbohydrates, it's normal and even expected to feel a bit of discomfort during the first few days of cutting back. You might find yourself missing these foods and craving them with a startling intensity, but there are some ways you can distract yourself enough to move past this initial phase of withdrawal.

- **Get plenty of fiber and fat.** Together, these foods can provide your body with some much-needed satiety. Flax seeds are a great option to get both of these at once, or salads with a lean protein added.

- **Snack frequently.** Don't go more than three hours without eating a healthy, low-carb snack, especially during your withdrawal from carbs. If you can avoid being hungry, you'll have better luck fighting cravings.

- **Find things you want to eat.** This diet is strict, but there are still tons of delicious things you can eat on an Atkins diet. Discover approved foods that you'll look forward to eating so your body will begin to crave those healthy alternatives, instead of carbohydrates.

- Do something for yourself. You're making a great change to improve your well-being, so instead of indulging in an unhealthy craving, do something else you enjoy. Read a book, take a bubble bath, or turn to a loved one for some support and encouragement.

Even once you're out of that initial withdrawal phase, some people experience a second period of "carb crash" where they have reported symptoms of feeling "off." Some people feel jittery or shaky, some feel fatigued, and some feel irritable. These symptoms will disappear after a couple of days, but you can try to prevent them from being overwhelming by indulging in a serving of low-carb fruit.

This can also be caused by a lack of salt, since many people on the Atkins diet will lose quite a bit of water weight within the first few days – which means a loss of sodium. If low-carb fruit doesn't help relieve the symptoms, try drinking a cup of bouillon a few times a day – and ensure that you are getting plenty of potassium.

You're going to have to learn to count carbs.

This sounds a lot more intimidating than it is, but there is definitely a learning curve involved with carb counting. The more you do it, the easier it will get – but in the beginning, a trip to the grocery store will be a little more involved than you're probably used to.

Since the induction phase of the Atkins diet has a strict requirement of under 20 grams of carbs each day, you will need to read food labels carefully to make sure you stay under your carb limit. Once you've passed this stage, you will be able to add more low-carb foods to your diet, and eventually reach a point where you can consume as many healthy carbs as your body can handle without gaining weight – but you'll always need to be thinking about what's in the foods you're eating.

When reading product labels, be sure to check the serving size as well as the carbohydrate count. If you are going to be eating more of a specific food, you may need to double or triple the total carbohydrate number in order to get an accurate estimate of what your intake will be.

Some people find it easier to count carbs by tracking each meal on an app that gives a breakdown of the nutritional content of your daily food intake. This way, you'll be able to clearly see how much carbohydrate is in the foods you eat, and then you can make the necessary adjustments to stay within the recommended range.

Eating an Atkins diet is time consuming.

If you're the kind of person who usually grabs food on the go, you'll have to make some big changes in order to adjust to an Atkins-style diet. It's hard to find readily available foods that will fit the restrictions of this diet, so be prepared to either make most of your meals yourself, or ask for modified versions of foods on most restaurant menus.

Even grocery shopping will take longer initially, as you learn about carbohydrates and calculate how much of each food you'll be able to eat. This will get easier with time, though, and soon you'll be able to hit the store and get what you need without a second thought.

You'll also be spending more time in the kitchen, prepping meals and cooking for yourself or for your family. If you have more free time on the weekends, you can always do the prep work in advance and come home to heat up pre-portioned servings of Atkins-approved meals. This is a great way to teach yourself to cook and learn your way around the kitchen, though, and like carb counting, it will get easier with practice.

This diet is a lifestyle change.

Eating an Atkins diet isn't just about losing weight – it's about making valuable changes to your entire lifestyle to achieve long-term health benefits. Sure, you'll probably see fat loss and watch the number on the scale go down, but in order to maintain these results, you'll need to look at Atkins as a lifestyle commitment.

Surrounding yourself with supportive people is a great way to ensure you can stick to this diet and make it a life-long habit. It might be difficult at first, to go out for dinner and drinks with friends and stick to Atkins-approved choices, but if you're with people who want to see you succeed, you'll be able to keep your social commitments while sticking to your Atkins diet.

Also, you might want to pack healthy, approved snacks for instances where other people are snacking around you – like when someone brings donuts or chips to the office, or at a party with tons of processed junk foods. If you have something quick and easy on-hand to snack on instead of indulging in the foods you've worked hard to avoid, you won't be nearly as tempted to cheat on your healthy new lifestyle.

How can I get started?

If you normally eat a diet that includes a variety of carbohydrates, making the switch to a diet like Atkins can be pretty intimidating. A good rule to keep in mind is to stick to unprocessed, natural, whole foods as much as you can. This will help you limit your intake of foods that aren't included on your diet plan without having to spend too much time thinking about it.

Take the list of approved Atkins foods to the grocery store and pick up everything you need to get started with these low-carb meal options. These recipes will help you get started on your journey to Atkins-style eating, helping you lose weight and achieve a wide range of important health benefits.

Keep in mind that most of your shopping should happen along the outside edges of the store – most of the aisles are full of processed foods.

As you practice making these Atkins-friendly meals, you'll learn more about low-carb eating and start coming up with your own inspired recipes. Hopefully your journey to healthier eating will help you discover new foods you didn't even know you liked, and motivate you to maintain your beneficial Atkins lifestyle.

Chapter 3:
The Phases Of The Atkins Diet
Four Phases

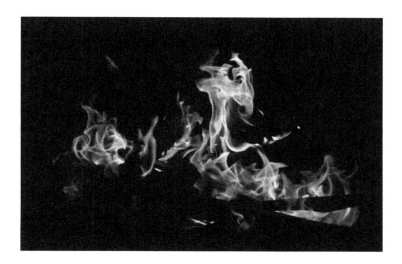

The Atkins diet has four phases:

Phase 1 – Induction

What You Eat On in The Induction Phase

From day one on Induction – you can eat all types of meat, fish, shellfish as well as a huge range of salads and vegetables. You will notice that there are no carbs in meat and fish while the number of net carbs in the vegetables in phase one are quite low. In the Induction phase, 12- 15g of your daily carbs should come from the foundation vegetables listed under phase one.

The next step is to turn lists of food into meals. We found the easiest approach for the first two weeks was to simply follow the meal plans at the back of the New Atkins New You book. Alternatively, the Starter Box comes with a Quick Start Guide with a two-week meal plan. Another option is the meal planner on the Atkins site – it has hundreds of meals to choose from so whatever your preferences and tastes you will be able to put together a meal plan to suit you – check out the Atkins recipes here or click on 'Create your plan' on this page. The foods you get to eat on Atkins from day one really are delicious so prepare to enjoy!

The advantage of following one of the meal plans above is that the carbs are already calculated for each meal and add up to the recommended 20g per day. Feel free to repeat meals you like or substitute other vegetables, side dishes, snacks or desserts as desired as long as the carb counts are comparable. To check how many carbs are in a food just check the Acceptable Food List. You receive a carb counter book in your Starter Box which includes a comprehensive list of foods and their carb counts.

As you get used to counting carbs, it is a good idea to experiment with different recipes to make sure you find meals that will suit your tastes, budget, time constraints etc. After all, you will not stick to this way of eating if you don't like the food so it's worth putting in the effort to make sure you do customize it to your tastes and lifestyle. The New Atkins New You book has lots of tips to help everyone to follow this program no matter what your culinary preferences, whether you eat out a lot or whether you are vegetarian or vegan!

What is off limits?

The part that everyone thinks is going to be the most difficult with the Atkins diet is the idea of giving up bread, baked products and foods like pasta. You probably won't believe this now but once you stop eating high carb foods like this, you also stop craving them! So for Paul and I, passing up on a slice of toast or a scone is no act of will-power, we simply don't want them anymore. And this kicks in very quickly – after two weeks or even less. So for now just take our word for it – it is much easier than you think it will be! Also it really is better if you do not cheat on this because if you do, you will just start the cravings all over again. So here is a list of what is off limits in Induction:

- Caloric fizzy drinks
- Fruits and fruit juices (other than lemon and lime juice and any fruits listed on the Acceptable Food List)
- Foods made with flour or other grain products – bread, cereal, pasta, muffins, scones, biscuits, crisps, cakes and products like gravy and packet mixes which usually contain flour
- Sugar, sweets and any foods containing added sugar – check the carb amounts on the label.
- Junk food in any form.
- Grains – even whole grains, rice, oats, barley etc.
- Alcohol (but don't worry you can re-introduce it in a few weeks' time in Phase 2)
- Any vegetables not on the Acceptable Food List including starchy vegetables like potatoes, carrots and parsnips. Don't worry however – there is a list of more than 50 other vegetables you can eat!
- On Induction you can eat dairy products such as cream, sour cream, butter and the hard cheeses listed on the Acceptable Food List. However other dairy products including milk (especially low-fat or skimmed milk), cottage cheese, ricotta or yoghurt are off-limits.
- 'Low-fat' foods or 'diet' products – they are usually surprisingly high in carbohydrates so steer clear.
- Any foods with manufactured trans-fats – this may be listed as hydrogenated or partially-hydrogenated oils.

The list above is not a complete list but use your common sense and stick to the Acceptable Food List and you'll be fine. Also if you have any questions, just ask your Atkins Support Partner .

Top Tips for Induction

The top tips for Induction are:

- Take some time to plan your meals for week one. This way of eating may be quite different from what you are used to so give yourself some time to prepare. This way of eating will become second nature in no time but it is going to require some extra time and effort at the beginning.
- Although you will probably find you are eating more vegetables than you did previously, it is recommended that you take a daily multivitamin and an omeaga-3 fatty acid supplement.
- Buy a notebook and write down what you eat and the amount of carbs at least for the first few weeks. We all selectively remember what we did (or didn't eat!) otherwise. Believe me, this step alone will make a big difference.
- Take a photo before you start. Wear something figures hugging and take a side and front profile pic. You will be so glad you did in a few weeks or months' time when you can compare photos from then with the 'before' picture and see your progress. Also take your measurements – you'll find a measuring tape in your Starter Box. This is important because sometimes you will see the difference in inches before you see it on the scales.
  The Starter Box also includes a weight and measurement tracker. The actual number on the scales is not important. You just need to know what it is so you can see what progress you've made in two weeks' time.
- One of the science based changes in the New Atkins is the recommendation to drink 2 cups of broth, half a teaspoon of salt or 2 tablespoons of regular soya sauce. For Irish readers, you might be familiar with Bovril. As with any diet, you will lose a certain amount of water at the beginning. For some, this can be too much of a good thing as it causes you to lose salts as well and for some people this can cause them to feel tired or weak or to

have headaches when they start the Atkins diet. Drinking 2 cups of Bovril will prevent these symptoms. And no this does not make Atkins a high sodium diet!

- Don't forget that sugar is off limits so remember to buy sweetener like sucralose (Splenda), saccharine (Sweet'N Low), stevia (Sweet Leaf or Truvia) or xylitol and have that in your tea or coffee instead of sugar (if you take sugar). Have no more than 3 packets a day and count each packet as 1g of carbs. Also a good idea to get one of the little containers to keep in your handbag (or pocket for the men?!). Most cafes will have sweetener however but still handy to have particularly when visiting friends.

- Milk including skimmed milk is naturally rich in milk sugar (lactose) so its off-limits in Induction. However, cream is an acceptable and delicious alternative in tea/coffee! Just buy fresh cream or double cream – it really is lovely – and once you try it you'll never want to go back!

- Eat 3 meals and 2 snacks every day. Don't skip meals or go more than 6 waking hours without eating. You should definitely not be hungry on this diet!

- Drink lots of water.

- Don't forget to stock up on your Atkins products so you have suitable snacks to hand at all times. Keep them in your desk at work, your car, handbag – that way you always have a healthy low carb option to hand – they are particularly good if you are out-and-about or busy. You can have two products a day and you certainly will not feel deprived when eating snacks like the delicious Chocolate Chip Daybreak bar or the Advantage Chocolate Crunch bar or the like! The shakes are delicious and very convenient as well. As well as tasting good, the bars (especially the Advantage range) are very filling so they will fill you up and stop you for reaching for unsuitable high-carb alternatives.

- Check the amount of carbohydrates on labels of everything you buy – don't assume anything is low in carbs. In Ireland, you can just go by the total amount of carbohydrates on the label (on the Atkins site you may see comments about deducting fiber from the carb amount – this is because the labeling is different in the US and includes fiber in the carbohydrate count). However, you will probably find you are buying much less food that comes with labels with this way of eating in any case i.e. meat, poultry, fish and vegetables.

By starting the Atkins diet, you are embarking on a journey that will make a huge difference to your health and well-being – congratulations for taking that first step! Your Atkins Support Partner is there to help you, so be sure to take advantage of that.

Phase 2 – Ongoing Weight Loss

Phase 2 is also called Ongoing Weight Loss or **OWL**. Most people spend the majority of their weight loss time in this phase. Initially the differences between Induction and OWL are very small. In OWL, the idea is that you gradually reintroduce other carbohydrate foods bit by bit, while continuing to lose weight.

- Gradually add carbohydrates in the form of nutrient-dense foods, increasing to 25 grams of Net Carbs per day the first week, and moving up each week or every several weeks by 5-gram increments until weight loss stops.
- Continue to stay in control of your appetite and lose weight.
- Find your Carbohydrate Level for Losing (CLL) i.e. the amount of carbohydrates you can eat each day and continue to lose weight.

MOVING ON.

It is really important that you do move into OWL and you do not stay in Induction until you have reached your goal weight. The reason for this is so that you find out what foods you can eat, whether there are carbohydrate foods you are intolerant to and get closer to what will be a permanent way of eating so you maintain your goal weight once you reach it. By the end of OWL you will have an individualized eating plan – it is based on what you have discovered during this process works for you and your body. This is all geared towards making sure that once you have lost the extra weight, it stays lost!

The Carb Ladder

The following carb ladder shows you the order in which you re-introduce carbohydrate foods in OWL. You will already be eating the foods from Rung 1 and Rung 2 from Induction (if you started in Induction). You reintroduce the other foods starting with Rung 3 in Phase 2:

Rung 1: Foundation vegetables – leafy greens and other low-carb vegetables

Rung 2: Dairy foods low in carbs – cream, sour cream and most hard cheeses

Rung 3: Nuts and seeds including nut and seed butters.

Rung 4: Berries, cherries and melon (not watermelon).

Rung 5: Whole milk yoghurt and fresh cheeses, such as cottage cheese and ricotta.

Rung 6: Legumes, including chickpeas, lentils, edamame and the like.

Rung 7: Tomato and vegetable juice "cocktail" and more lemon and lime juice.

Rung 8: Other fruits (not fruit juices or dried fruits)

Rung 9: Starchy vegetables such as winter squash, carrots, peas in pods

Rung 10: Whole grains (not refined grain products)

The foods on the lower rungs are the foods you should be eating most often. On the top rungs are foods that will put in an appearance only occasionally, rarely or never depending on your carb tolerance. So as you can see from the carb ladder and the Atkins food pyramid below you will continue to eat a variety of meat, fish & poultry as well as an abundance of vegetables as well as including healthy fats.

Tips for Success

One important point to keep in mind with OWL is that you will be increasing the range of food you eat in OWL but does does not mean you will be increasing the amount by very much. As with Induction, you should definitely not be hungry so let your appetite be your guide.

The best way to do OWL is to introduce one new food from a group at a time. So for instance you might move on to berries and start by eating a small portion of blueberries. Assuming they cause no problems, you could move on to strawberries in a day or two. What you want to look out for and pay attention to is whether the new food reawakens food cravings, causes gastric distress or interferes with your weight loss. If a food does cause any problems, you can just leave it out and try re-introducing it at a later stage.

If you have been estimating carb counts, now is the time to start counting them. We would recommend that you write down what you eat each day along with the carb counts. That way you will know exactly where you are and it will make it easy to identify if there is a particular food that reawakens cravings or interferes with your weight-loss or causes any other health issues. Ordinarily most of us don't pay enough attention to how we feel and what foods might have caused this but this is a great opportunity to do just that and keeping a food diary and introducing foods one by one makes it much easier.

Now that you are in Phase 2 you can eat all of the convenient and delicious Atkins products including the delicious Endulge bars like the Endulge Chocolate Crisp, Endulge Peanut Caramel and the Endulge Coconut bar. Make sure that you have your Advantage or Daybreak bars or shakes on hand when you are out and about so that you don't resort to eating inappropriate high carb foods.

Phase 3 – Pre-Maintenance

By the time you move to Phase 3, you will be close to achieving your goal weight with just 10 pounds to go. You will also have identified foods that your body can or cannot handle as well as the amount of carbohydrates you can eat daily and continue losing weight. You will almost certainly have noticed other health benefits and improvements in general well-being by now as well. Congratulations!

Phase 3 continues this important process of learning exactly what you need to know to make sure the weight stays lost and you maintain the slim new you. So the objectives of the Pre-Maintenance phase are:

Lose the last 10 pounds slowly – it is tempting to want to get to your goal weight as quickly as possible but its important that you do slow it down as you move towards a permanent way of eating. It may take several months to reach your goal weight, losing perhaps just half a pound a week. Those last few pounds and centimeters can be the most stubborn so it is normal for it to slow down at this stage. If you rush to lose those last few pounds you may never learn what you need to know to keep them off for good..

Test your carb tolerance – as you slow down your weight loss you may be able to increase your Carbohydrate Level for Losing (CLL). The CLL was the number you discovered at the end of Phase 2 – the amount of grams of carbs you can eat each day and continue to lose weight. Now that you are slowing down the weight loss and moving to weight maintenance, you may be able to increase this number.

- Test your tolerance for additional foods – as in Phase 2 you can re-introduce whole food carbohydrates and note how they make you feel. These will be foods at the top of the carbohydrate ladder (see below) like fruit higher in carbs, starchy veg and unprocessed whole grains. It is important to pay attention to how you feel when you introduce new foods. For example, it they cause cravings to come back or any other adverse effects on your health or well-being it's best to eliminate them. And fantastic that you have discovered this – many people go through life eating foods they are intolerant to and suffering the effects of this.

- Find your ACE (Atkins Carbohydrate Equilibrium) – this is the number of grams of carbs you can eat daily and neither gain or lose weight. This is the magic number that will help you stay at your goal weight – forever! Ideally, you want to reach your ACE level when you're at your goal weight. So, adjust your carbs as needed to keep losing if you're not there yet. Many people end up with an ACE of between 65 and 100 grams of carbs. Some people might be considerably less and a few others could even higher.

- Maintain your control and your weight. Once you have found your ACE and before you move to phase 4 – Lifetime Maintenance – maintain your weight for a month. You can continue to introduce new foods once you don't go over your ACE. Again, pay close attention to how these new foods affect you if at all. This month is really the dress rehearsal for the Lifetime Maintenance phase.

How to do Phase 3 – Pre-Maintenance

- Add 10g of daily carbs every week or every few weeks. If you finished Phase 2 at with a CLL (Carbohydrate Level for Losing) of 45 grams of carbs, start Phase 3 with 55 grams of carbs a day. Then increase your daily carb intake every week or every few weeks by 10 grams. If weight loss stalls or cravings return step back by 10g.

- Count carbs – you have probably gathered from the objectives above that you will need to write down what you eat and note the carb amounts. Otherwise you will really know how many grams of carbs you are eating and will not be able to discover your ACE. Again this will also let you identify easily if a new food is causing a problem.

- As you have done from the beginning, be sure that at least 12 to 15 grams of your total daily carb intake is made up of foundation vegetables – see the veg in Phase 1 of the Acceptable Food List for a list of over 50 of these along with tips on how to cook them and links to recipes.
- Add new foods one by one, following the Carb Ladder, starting with legumes, unless you've been able to reintroduce them in OWL—as vegetarians and vegans almost certainly have.
- Keep eating the recommended amounts of protein and sufficient natural fats to feel satisfied at the end of each meal.
- Continue to drink plenty of water and other acceptable beverages.
- Consume enough salt, broth, or soy sauce (unless you take diuretics) to avoid symptoms that may accompany the switch to fat-burning as long as your Net Carb intake is 50 grams or less. Two cups of Bovril a day will do the trick also. Once you exceed 50 grams of carbs this you won't need this.
- Take your multivitamin/multi mineral and omega-3 fatty acid supplements.
- Be sure to have your Atkins bars, shakes and treats on hand to prevent you from resorting to bad choices that might derail your progress.

What happens if I reach a plateau?

There's a good chance that at some point you reach a plateau and stop losing weight. The pace of weight loss is often erratic and many people lose weight in fits and starts. However, the definition of a plateau when you lose nothing despite doing everything for a period of at least four weeks. If you are losing centimeters but not weight, then this is not a true plateau and you should keep doing what you are doing. Hitting a plateau can be very frustrating but dealing patiently with it is crucial to your continued success. Try the following tips:

- Tighten up on recording everything you eat and the carb amounts – this can make a big difference.
- Count all your carbs including lemon juice, sweetners etc
- Decrease your daily intake of carbs by 10 grams. You may simply have stumbled on your ACE (i.e. the number of grams of carbs or maintaining your weight) early. Once weight loss resumes move up in 5 gram increments again.
- Find and eliminate hidden carbs in sauces, drinks and processed foods.
- Increase your activity level or try new activities – this works for some people but not all.
- Increase your fluid intake to at least 8 glasses of water a day.
- Cut back on artificial sweeteners, low-carb products and fruits other than berries.

Check your calorie intake. We do not usually count calories on Atkins but if you are doing everything to the letter and haven't lost weight in 4 weeks you may need to check your calories. You probably could guess that too many calories will slow down your weight loss, but here's a surprise—too few will slow down your metabolism and slow weight loss. The numbers will vary depending on your height, age and metabolism but it should be within the following ranges:

- Women: 1,500–1,800 calories a day.
- Men: 1,800–2,000 calories per day.

If you've been consuming alcohol, cut back or abstain for now.

If none of these modifications makes the scales budge for a month, then you really are on a plateau. The only way to overcome it is to continue to eat right and wait. Your body and the scales will eventually comply.

Tips for Success

The top tip for success is to have patience and follow the process. Also remember why you want to lose weight and improve your health – write down your reasons if it helps. Doing this will get you to your goal weight and mean you know what you need in order to stay there. permanently!

Phase 4 – Maintenance

Congratulations! You have reached your ideal weight! It's a fantastic achievement – and a position that many many people who are overweight would like to be in. I'm sure clothes shopping or beach holidays are much more fun now! And hearing positive comments from people you haven't seen in a while!

You can be sure that your health markers are all telling a positive story too – if you had a check up before you started now would be a great time to do it again to see exactly how much those numbers have improved. You might well find that if you were on medication for high blood pressure, cholesterol or other conditions that these are no longer needed – check with your doctor. If you are diabetic, you should have been closely monitored by your doctor during this journey and have possibly already reduced if not eliminated your medications under their guidance. If you think back to before you started this journey, you have probably noticed many minor ailments or some not so minor have disappeared along this journey to the slim healthy new you.

Here are just some of the benefits that you need to know for the atkins diet phase 4:

- Improved cholesterol
- Lower triglycerides (these are a marker for heart disease)
- One diabetic reported blood sugar dropping from 7.9 to 3.9 – which is in the normal range
- Sleeping better
- Migraines gone

- Acne cleared up
- Painkillers not needed for PMS anymore
- Acid reflux gone – had been on 2 tablets a day for 15 years
- Bloated feeling after meals gone
- 'Mental fog' gone
- More energy
- No longer needs a nap in the afternoon
- Joint pain gone
- Improved self-esteem

Of course, these improvements often lead to improvements in other areas of life and business too. Many of these benefits kicked a mere week or two after starting Induction. However, human nature being what it is we tend to forget it after a while and feeling this good becomes the new normal, as it should. Now that you have reached Maintenance it is worth taking stock and thinking back on all the benefits you have gained with this way of life – both in terms of weight loss, health, vitality and general feel-good factor. This will help you with staying on this path and maintaining all of these benefits.

HOW TO DO PHASE 4 – MAINTENANCE

In Pre-Maintenance you learned what your ACE (Atkins Carbohydrate Equilibrium) was– this is the number of grams of carbs you can eat daily and neither gain or lose weight. All you need to do is continue to eat the way you've been eating in Pre-Maintenance, remaining at or just below your ACE.

For those with a high ACE:

If you have a high carbohydrate threshold and are physically active you are already eating foods from rungs 7 – 10 of the carbohydrate ladder. These would include starchy vegetables, fruit other than berries and whole grains – see the Atkins Carb ladder for more. As before when you introduce new foods, pay attention to how they make you feel and whether they weight gain, hunger or cause cravings to come back.

For those with an ACE below 50g:

If your carbohydrate threshold is below 50 grams of Net Carbs, you'll probably have to stay away from starchy vegetables, most fruit and whole grains or eat them rarely or in very small amounts. Exercising is one excellent way to increase you carbohydrate level and many people feel much more inclined to do so after they have lost some weight and have increased energy levels. Even if it turns out that your ACE is quite low – it's important to keep in mind that at least now you know what you need in order to maintain your weight and keep all those benefits we spoke about. After all the goal is to banish that extra weight forever – not win a competition for having the highest ACE possible!

You also know at this stage that there are lots of delicious meals you can enjoy no matter what your ACE. And as only someone who has followed this nutritional approach can understand, you know that giving up those refined carbs you used to eat for good is not at all a difficult prospect you imagined before beginning this way of eating. So it really is fantastic that you have learned what you need to stay slim and healthy forever – whatever the carb level.

What You Can Eat in Phase 4

In the Maintenance Phase your level of carbohydrates will essentially be the same as it was in Pre-Maintenance. Of course, you can re-introduce new foods in the months and years to come while staying below that carbohydrate level – as before be alert to see whether they cause weight gain or any other adverse effects.

Many people find that their appetite increases slightly as they approach their body's natural healthy weight even as they stay within their ACE. Now that you are no longer burning body fat for fuel it's important to understand that the extra fuel to keep your weight stable should come from dietary fat instead. In this way, your body stays in fat-burning mode. This is important so that you don't veer back to a state where your body burns carbs as it primary fuel – which brings back those blood sugar swings, poor energy and inevitably weight-gain. So if your weight drops below the desired level or you find that you are hungry you should also slightly increase good fats in your diet. To give you some ideas, you could add 3 – 5 portions of the following (as your appetite dictates) to your diet:

- 1 tablespoon of oil for dressing salads
- 1 tablespoon of butter
- 2 tablespoons of cream
- 5g cheese
- 10 large ripe olives with a teaspoon of olive oil
- Half an advocado
- 30g of almonds, walnuts, pecans or macadamias
- 1 tablespoon of full fat mayonnaise
- 2 tablespoons of pesto
- 2 tablespoons of nut butter

Hopefully by now, you are no longer afraid of fats (as many people are due the the fat-phobic advice we're all been given over the last 30 years) and you know that dietary fat is good for you in the context of a low carbohydrate diet. Your body at this stage is a very efficient fat-burning machine and these additions of fat in your diet will help keep your weight stable (as counter-intuitive as this might sound). The only dietary fat you should truly avoid are trans fats. An increased intake of trans fats is associated with an increased heart attack risk and inflammation in the body. They are typically found in foods you should be avoiding already, including fried foods, baked goods, biscuits, crackers, sweets, snack foods, icings and vegetable shortenings.

Phase 4 And The Rest of Your Life

Hopefully you understand by now that you will remain on phase 4 – the Lifetime Maintenance Phase – for the rest of your life! This makes sure the weight you have so successfully lost, stays lost forever! As we've said from the outset this diet is more of a lifestyle change and way-of-eating for life than a 'diet' you follow for a few weeks or months and then stop. If you go back to the way you used to eat, you will get the results you got the first time – weight gain and all that goes with it.

Of course we are not saying that you can't ever eat a slice of cake or the occasional slice of pizza. In the same way that some people are fine with alcohol in moderation, some people will find they can have these foods occasionally and it doesn't cause any problems. However, for others having just a little is the same as someone that can't handle alcohol – they find it much easier to avoid it completely and that it's just not worth the chance of eating these foods leading to a full-blown binge.

It is important to arrive at a place where you are mindful of your weight but not obsessed with it. Keep an eye on your weight and your measurements. Be alert to cravings coming back, unreasonable hunger or the return of any symptoms you had banished. Then take a look at what you have been eating. Maybe it was a case of carb creep or the effects or one or two recently added foods. Never let yourself gain more than 5 lbs without taking action to restore your goal weight. If this happens simply drop 10 to 20g of carbs and the weight should retreat. Or if need be, return to OWL for a week or two under it is under control again.

Keep in mind too that life events can affect your weight and cause you to slip:

You used to play a team sport but had an injury and had to stop

You had a baby and find yourself stressed and sleep deprived

Your doctor prescribes anti-depressants to help you deal with a family crisis

A new job means you need to travel more making it more difficult to keep up with you fitness regime and plan suitable meals

You suffer a disappointment or a break-up and this sends you back to your old unhealthy eating habits

You start a new relationship with someone who doesn't follow the Atkins diet

The key in all of these situations is to be mindful of these life changes and make adjustments to remain at your desired weight. There are lots of strategies you can take to deal with different life events so they don't derail the fantastic progress you've made and so that you achieve the ultimate goal of staying slim.

Chapter 4:
Food List Of The Atkins Diet

If you're giving the Atkins diet a try, then you need to add these foods to your grocery list.

Atkins Diet List of Foods

If you're having trouble finding out what to make for dinner, there are plenty of Atkins diet recipes online and in print that include acceptable Atkins diet snacks and Atkins diet desserts. Don't have the time to find Atkins diet meal plans yourself? Just download the app for quick access to hundreds of daily meal options. Although there are several Atkins diet recipes on the actual Atkins site, here is a comprehensive list of all of the foods you can eat on the Atkins 20 Atkins diet plan.

Atkins Diet Phase 1

The Atkins diet Phase 1 (also known as the "induction" phase) list of acceptable foods includes:

- All fish, including: flounder, sole, herring, salmon, sardines, tuna, trout, cod, halibut.
- All fowl, including: Cornish hen, chicken, duck, goose, pheasant, quail, turkey, and ostrich.
- All shellfish, including: clams, crabmeat, mussels, oysters, shrimp, squid, and lobster. (Please note that oysters and mussels are higher in carbs, so if you're craving either, you should limit yourself to four ounces per day.)
- All meat, including: bacon, beef, ham, lamb, pork, veal, and venison. (Please note that some processed meats, like bacon and ham, are cured with sugar. Check the package before indulging!)

- Any egg prepared in any style, including: deviled, fried, hard boiled, omelets, poached, scrambled, and soft-boiled.
- Fats (the good kind) and oils, including: butter, mayonnaise (with no added sugar), olive oil, vegetable oils, canola oil, walnut oil, soybean oil, sesame oil, grape seed oil, sunflower oil, safflower oil.
- Artificial sweeteners, including: sucralose, saccharin, and stevia.
- Beverages including: clear broth, bouillon (make sure there's no sugar added), club soda, cream (heavy or light), decaffeinated or regular coffee and tea, diet soda (take note of the carb count, which should be zero), flavored seltzer (no-calorie seltzer only), herb tea (without added barley or fruit sugar), unflavored soy/almond milk, and water (eight ounces per day). Water options include filtered water, mineral water, spring water, and tap water.
- Cheese, including: Parmesan (grated), goat, cheddar, gouda, mozzarella (whole milk), cream cheese (whipped), Swiss, and feta. (Cheese is an amazing thing, but it does contain carbs, so you should stick to three to four ounces of cheese per day.)
- Foundation vegetables, including: alfalfa sprouts, chicory greens, endives, escaroles, olives (green and black), watercress, arugula, radishes, spinach, bok choy, lettuce, turnip greens, hearts of palm, radicchio, artichoke, celery, collard greens, pickles, broccoli rabe, sauerkraut, avocados, daikon radish, red and white onions, zucchini, cucumbers, cauliflower, beet greens, broccoli, fennel, okra, rhubarb, swiss chard, asparagus, broccolini, bell peppers, sprouts, eggplants, kale, scallions, turnips, tomatoes, jicama, portobello mushrooms, yellow squash, cabbage, green beans, leeks, shallots, brussel sprouts, cherry tomatoes, spaghetti squash, kohlrabi, pumpkin, snow peas, and garlic. (During Phase 1, you should be eating roughly 12 to 15 grams of net carbs per day in the form of vegetables. This

high-fat, high-protein, and low-carb introduction will give you a solid kick start.)

- Salad garnishes, including: crumbled bacon, hard-boiled egg, sauteed mushrooms, sour cream, and grated cheeses.
- Herbs and spices, including: basil, cayenne pepper, cilantro, dill, oregano, tarragon, parsley, chives, ginger, rosemary, sage, black pepper, and garlic.
- Salad dressings, including: red wine vinegar, caesar, ranch, lemon juice, blue cheese, lime juice, balsamic vinegar, Italian, and creamy Italian.

Atkins Diet Phase 2

Below is the Atkins diet Phase 2 (also known as the "Balancing" phase) list of acceptable foods (this list, plus the items listed above). You'll be allowed to add higher carbs into your diet during Phase 2 (think nuts and fruits).

- Dairy, including: mozzarella cheese, yogurt (Greek and plain), unsweetened milk, whole milk, ricotta cheese, cottage cheese, and heavy cream.
- Nuts and seeds, including: Brazil nuts, macadamias, hulled sunflower seeds, walnuts, almonds, pistachios, peanuts, pecans, and cashews.
- Fruits, including: blackberries, raspberries, cranberries, strawberries, cantaloupe, honeydew, gooseberries, boysenberries, and blueberries.
- Juices, including: lemon juice, lime juice, and tomato juice.
- Beans, including: lentils, kidney beans, lima beans, pinto beans, black beans, navy beans, great northern beans, and chickpeas.

Atkins Diet Phase 3

Below is the Atkins diet Phase 3 (also referred to as the "Fine-Tuning" phase) list of acceptable foods (this list, plus the items listed above):

- Starchy vegetables, including: carrots, rutabaga, beets, acorn squash, sweet potatoes, parsnips, potatoes, and corn.
- Fruit, including: coconut, figs, cherries, watermelon, pomegranate, papayas, plums, guava, apples, clementines, grapefruit, kiwis, apricots, pineapple, peaches, mangoes, grapes, oranges, dates, bananas, and pears.
- Grains, including: wheat bran, wheat germ, oat bran, quinoa, whole-wheat bread, oatmeal, polenta, grits, whole-wheat pasta, barley, millet, and rice.

Once you've reached Phase 4, you've learned which foods boost the metabolism and which foods you should avoid. All of the "acceptable" foods in the fourth phase of the Atkins diet overlap with the foods listed in Phase 3, so you shouldn't have any problem transitioning.

Atkins Diet Phase 4

Below is the Atkins diet Phase 4 (also known as the "Maintenance" phase) list of acceptable foods (this list, plus the items listed above):

- Starchy vegetables including: carrots, rutabaga, beets, peas, acorn squash, butternut squash, sweet potatoes, parsnips, potatoes, and corn.
- Fruit, including: coconuts, figs, cherries, watermelon, pomegranate seeds, papayas, plums, raisins, guava, clementines, apples, kiwis, grapefruit, apricots, pineapples, peaches, mangoes, grapes, oranges, dates, bananas, and pears.
- Grains, including: wheat bran, wheat germ, oat bran, quinoa, whole-wheat bread, oatmeal, polenta, grits, whole-wheat pasta, barley, millet, and rice.

Chapter 5:
Breakfast Recipes

ALMOND AND COCONUT MUFFIN

Ingredients

- 2 tablespoons Almond Meal Flour
- 1 teaspoon Coconut flour, high fiber
- 1 teaspoon Sucralose Based Sweetener (Sugar Substitute)
- 1/2 teaspoon Cinnamon
- 1/4 teaspoon Baking Powder (Straight Phosphate, Double Acting)
- 1/8 teaspoon Salt
- 1 large Egg
- 1 teaspoon Extra Virgin Olive Oil
- 1 tablespoon Sour Cream

Instructions

1) Place all dry ingredients in a coffee mug. Stir to combine.
2) Add the egg, oil, and sour cream. Stir until thoroughly combined.
3) Microwave for 1 minute. Use a knife if necessary to help remove the muffin from the cup, slice, butter, eat. For best results, eat immediately.

Note: Almond Meal from whole almonds is preferred for this recipe. Your MIM can be toasted once it's cooked and topped with cream cheese if you like. Replace the cinnamon with other spices, sugar-free syrup or 1/2 tsp unsweetened cocoa (net carb count will be .2g higher). Change the shape by making it in a bowl.

ALMOND-PINEAPPLE SMOOTHIE

INGREDIENTS

- 1/2 cup (8 fluid ounces) Plain Yogurt (Whole Milk)
- 2 1/2 ounces Pineapple
- 20 each wholes Blanched & Slivered Almonds
- 1/2 cup Pure Almond Milk - Unsweetened Original

INSTRUCTIONS

Feel free to substitute other fruits or nuts for the pineapple and/or almonds (about 20 whole almonds, 3 Tbsp slivered). Be sure to use fresh pineapple in this smoothie. Canned pineapple is swimming in sugar.

Combine the yogurt, pineapple, almonds and almond milk in a blender and purée until smooth and creamy.

ATKINS PANCAKES

INGREDIENTS

- 1 individual packet Sucralose Based Sweetener (Sugar Substitute)
- 2 teaspoons Baking Powder (Straight Phosphate, Double Acting)
- 1/4 teaspoon Salt
- 1 large Egg (Whole)
- 1 cup Cream (Half & Half)
- 3 servings Atkins Flour Mix

INSTRUCTIONS

Blend together 1 cup baking mix, sugar substitute, baking powder and salt in a large mixing bowl.

Add the half and half and egg. Whisk batter. Let the mixture sit for at least 5 minutes to activate the baking powder.

Coat the griddle with olive oil spray. Over medium heat, cook 4 pancakes at a time. When bubbles appear on the top and the edges are firm, flip the pancakes and cook another 2-3 minutes. Keep warm in the oven.

Repeat with remaining pancakes.

BAKED EGGS AND ASPARAGUS

- 8 spear, small (5" long or less) Asparagus
- 1/4 cup Heavy Cream
- 2 large Eggs (Whole)
- 2 tablespoons Almond Meal Flour
- 1 tablespoon Parmesan Cheese (Shredded)
- 1/8 teaspoon Garlic
- 1/8 teaspoon Black Pepper

INSTRUCTIONS

Preheat oven to 400°F. Prepare a small oven safe casserole or 4-inch by 3-inch dish with a little bit of oil. Set aside.

Boil the asparagus spears for 2 minutes until tender-crisp. Drain and run under cold water then pat dry. Arrange in the prepared baking dish.

Pour cream over the asparagus and then crack two eggs on top.

In a small bowl blend together the almond meal, Parmesan cheese, garlic and black pepper. Sprinkle over the eggs and place in the oven. Cook for 5-10 minutes depending upon how you like your eggs cooked. Longer time will result in a firmer yolk. The cream will puff over the edges of the eggs and the topping should be golden brown and fragrant.

ATKINS WAFFLES

INGREDIENTS

- 1 individual packet Sucralose Based Sweetener (Sugar Substitute)
- 1 large Egg (Whole)
- 2 teaspoons Baking Powder (Straight Phosphate, Double Acting)
- 1/4 teaspoon Salt
- 1 cup Cream (Half & Half)
- 3 servings Atkins Flour Mix

INSTRUCTIONS

Use the Atkins recipe to make Atkins Flour Mix for this recipe. This recipe makes 5 waffles. Assuming your waffle iron makes 4 servings, use four-fifths of the batter and then make a single waffle with the remaining batter. Freeze extra waffles and just pop in the toaster before serving.

In a large bowl, blend together 1 cup baking mix, baking powder, sugar substitute and salt. In another large bowl, mix the half-and-half and beaten egg.

Add dry ingredients to the liquid ingredients and whisk batter until any lumps are removed. Don't overbeat.

Let the mixture sit for at least 5 minutes to activate the baking powder.

Heat the waffle iron and pour the batter in the center of the waffle iron.

Close the top and cook waffles for about 1 1/2 minutes or until golden brown.

Repeat with last waffle.

BONUS CHAPTERS:

INTUITIVE EATING

Introduction

If you could profit every diet just like a frequent flyer program, the majority of us could have earned a vacation to the moon and back. The almost $60 billion at 12 months, the weight-loss industry could finance the trip for generations to arrive (Bacon and Aphramor 2011). Ironically, we appear to have significantly more respect for our vehicles than for ourselves. If you took your vehicle to a car mechanic for regular tune-ups, and after money and time spent, the automobile didn't function, and you wouldn't blame yourself. Yet, regardless of the fact that 90 to 95 per cent of most diets fail-you have a tendency to blame yourself, not the dietary plan! Isn't it ironic that with an enormous failure price for dieting-we don't blame the procedure of dieting?

Initially, whenever we ventured into the globe of private practice, we didn't know each other. Yet, separately, each folk had remarkably similar guidance experiences that triggered us to rethink how exactly we work. This resulted in a significant change in how exactly we practice and years, later on, was the impetus because of this book.

My objective for Intuitive eating wasn't fame or fortune, however. When I sat right down to write the book, I simply wished to educate and motivate visitors to achieve superior health, whether they wished to lose weight, feel good, or invert a chronic disease. I experienced no idea the publication would take off, or that it could resonate so deeply with people all over the world. It seemed everyone began using that phrase-intuitive eating-to explain the overwhelmingly effective eating design detailed in reserve. And to this full-day, there are apparently never-ending blasts of discussions, describing miraculous health adjustments, caused by this topic.

The trick behind Intuitive eating's popularity is easy: It didn't promise an instant fix. Unlike crash diets that guarantee easy and instant results, "Intuitive eating" organized vital details about food and healthful eating that allowed visitors to be specialists in nutrition. The publication essentially paid to its visitors the keys to effective weight reduction so that these were in charge of their health destiny.

Center to Intuitive eating is a straightforward health equation, the core idea of my nutritarian program:

H = N / C Wellness = Nutrients / Calories

Your wellbeing is predicted by your nutrient intake divided by your calorie consumption.

I contact this core idea the nutrient density of your daily diet. Food gives us nutrition and calorie consumption (energy). All calories result from only three components: carbohydrates, fat, and proteins. Nutrients, however, come from noncaloric food factors, namely, vitamin supplements, nutrients, fibres, and phytochemicals, actually chemical substances that generally occur in plants. These noncaloric nutrients are quite crucial to your wellbeing. When the ratio of nutrition to calorie consumption is high, fat burns up, and wellness is restored. The even more nutrient-dense meals you consume, the, even more, you'll be happy with fewer calories, and the much less you'll crave excess fat and high-calorie foods.

A high-nutrient diet decreases growing older, helps restoration cells, reduces inflammation, and helps rid your body of toxins. High-nutrient, low-calorie foods include a great deal of dietary fibre and take up a whole lot of space in the stomach. As you consume a more substantial quantity of food, it satiates your food cravings and blunts your hunger. Meeting the body's micronutrient requirements also helps suppress food craving and what I contact "toxic hunger, " which drives you to consume more calories than you require-usually in the type of processed foods, which can result in cancer and heart disease, among a great many other ailments.

Witnessing how Intuitive consuming inspired a lot of people to improve their diets not merely reinforced my results that high-nutrient diets create good wellness; it offered a considerable, ongoing body of proof proving that approach works. Nothing displays the energy of this method of consuming more than hearing from individuals who apply this understanding and live it each day in their personal lives. Thousands of individuals lost dramatic levels of weight without problems rather than regained it. One reader called Scott weighed an astounding 500 pounds. Scott couldn't tie his very own sneakers. His breathing was laboured, and he could walk only nine actions at a time. He was thirty-eight years aged. A doctor informed him that if he didn't undergo belly reduction surgery, he'd probably die within half a year. Scott spurned his doctor's guidance and instead made a decision to switch how he considered food and his method of eating by pursuing my high-nutrient meal strategy, which offered him with the nutrients, protein, and vitamin supplements he had a need to achieve good wellness. Because he right now eats for health, he can eat just as much as he wants, ignoring the scale fully. Today, Scott weighs 180 pounds and wants to exercise-a big differ from when he could not walk.

My individuals routinely lose up to 20 pounds through the first six weeks of changing their diet plan. And that's simply the start. More importantly, they typically get over diseases such as for example allergies, asthma, acne, headaches, high blood circulation pressure, diabetes, reflux esophagitis, lupus, kidney insufficiency, psoriasis, angina, cardiomyopathy, and multiple sclerosis-and they steadily get to get rid of their dependence on prescription drugs.

Though I have very long studied and utilized high- nutrient eating as a medical prescription for days gone by twenty-five years, actually I must admit to being amazed by a few of the phenomenal recoveries folks have reported if you ask me. Once, somebody asked whether this micronutrient-rich approach could change their hair back again to brownish from grey. "Of program not really," I answered. But, affirmed, on my website discussion board, two different people commented that it experienced occurred to them. I couldn't believe it. Similarly, among my sufferers had hepatitis C prior to starting my eating design. I didn't believe this high-nutrient eating design would remedy his hepatitis contamination and liver injury; nevertheless, after some right time, his hepatitis C disappeared. I had to do it again the blood tests 3 x to believe it. Seeing such dramatic recoveries from what exactly is conventionally considered irreversible illnesses excited me, making me even more adamant that delicious method of eating can result in medical transformations for an incredible number of Americans.

The total results and success stories are astounding. They come from folks of different back again- grounds, from different age groups, and they all began their journeys for different factors. Yet what they talk about in common is all of them are now in excellent wellness. For most of the Intuitive eating's achievement; however, I quickly found realize that science-based details about nutrition only wasn't enough. With these details available to such a wide audience, why would a lot of people neglect to recognize there have to protect their valuable health insurance and lose weight? Why would they become unable and unready to change? Why would they like to reject unassailable, scientific, and significantly effective advice? I'll let you know why, due to the mind-boggling twin powers of meals preference and meals addiction.

Just like the classic victim, we actually grow to love things that kill us-in this case, unhealthy food. Unhealthy eating styles and meals addictions have both used control of our brains, and this dependence on certain foods is frequently as deadly as many other addictions.

The standard American diet plan (SAD) is eliminating us. Rather than providing us with these basic needs once and for all health, it has created a country where disease and persistent illness are believed to be unavoidable and just another organic consequence of ageing. Carrying excess fat is the primary reason behind type 2 diabetes; it accelerates atherosclerosis and death from cardiovascular disease. In just a matter of years, excess body weight is usually projected to overtake smoking as the root cause of loss of life in the USA. By enough time, most Americans reach age fifty, they are already addicted to prescription drugs, and almost fifty per cent of People in America still die of heart attacks and strokes. You don't need to be one of them. Twenty-eight million Americans have problems with the crippling discomfort of osteoarthritis. You do not have to be one of these. Thirty-five million Americans have problems with persistent headaches. You don't need to be one of them. You simply don't need to be sick.

Today, 475 million adults all over the world suffer from obesity. That's a 50 per cent increase since 1980. Simultaneously, the amount of over- excess weight adults is fast approaching 1 billion, plus some 200 million school-age kids are already overweight, which means almost 1. 7 billion individuals are either overweight or obese. One nearly 7 billion people!

 In the USA alone, about two-thirds of People in America are overweight, based on the National Institutes of Wellness (NIH). But this doesn't tell the complete story. Both NIH and the Globe Health Business define an "obese" person to possess a body mass index (BMI) of 25. This implies that a woman who is 5 feet 5 inches tall is considered a standard pounds at 150 pounds, and a guy whose 5 feet 10 inches tall is considered regular at 175 pounds. This man and female may carry between 20 and 30 pounds of disease- leading to excess fat around their waists. However, they would be considered healthy and match by today's standards. This is not accurate to look at a person with that very much fat normal or healthy. If you look at societies or groups of individuals who live longer than average, you'll discover average group BMIs between 18 and 22- nowhere close to the American regular of 25. For instance, the

Okinawa Centenarian Study-which examined a lot more than 1000 centenarians from Okinawa, Japan, over twenty-five years from the mid-1970s to 2001-found that the common BMI of the studied adults was 20.4; The Adventist Health Study-who follow a mainly vegan diet-found an identical result. This twelve-year prospective study of thirty-four thousand middle-aged and elderly Adventists without preexisting illnesses, no background of smoking, cardiovascular system disease, malignancy, or stroke exposed a primary positive relation between a lesser BMI and longevity. An Adventist with a BMI greater than 23 does experience a higher threat of premature death.

Just what exactly can we study from these studies? Based on the data, the utmost acceptable weight generates a BMI of around 22.5, not 25. This implies that the recommended healthful weight for a 5-foot-10-inches adult male is usually between 130 and 160 pounds, and for 5-foot-5-inches adult female is 108 to 135 pounds. That is a large difference from the suitable (not obese) American BMI of 25, which allows 150 pounds for a female and 175 pounds for a guy.

Based on the Okinawan and Adventist regular BMI, about 85 per cent of Americans are overweight, not really the 66 per cent based on the NIH. The common American is definitely heavier and sicker than she or he even realizes. All due to the typical American diet. Hardly anyone can get away its destructive effects. Why else would 90 per cent of everybody older than sixty-five be taking medicines to lessen his or her blood circulation pressure and/or cholesterol? The end result is this: In the event that you eat American meals, you will inevitably develop the illnesses common in America, you shall become overweight, and you will ultimately develop high blood circulation pressure and raised cholesterol (the signs of bloodstream vessel and cardiovascular disease), just like everyone else.

We now contemplate it normal to reduce youthful vigour inside our thirties, carry a supplementary 30 to 40 pounds, live with chronic illness inside our past due forties and fifties, and endure our final years completely reliant on others. But this is simply not normal. This is actually the consequence of a lifelong design of harmful living and misguided info. Instead of dreading deterioration and an increasing number of ailments and medications as we approach later years, we should anticipate enjoying an active existence well into our nineties. This might seem like an outrageous expectation because the majority of us spend eternity eating an unhealthy diet. Today even, too many folks continue to skip the connection between what we consume and how we experience emotionally and actually. Nor can we find out why it appears so difficult to remain at our youthful adult weight.

But it's not as well late.

A high-nutrient diet will certainly reduce your desire to have high-calorie, low-nutrient foods. Within weeks, your taste buds will change, and you'll weary in the processed foods you once believed you could by no means live without. You'll experience more satisfied consuming fewer calorie consumption than you were consuming before. The result is lasting health and long term weight loss. So a lot of my visitors have dropped 100 pounds or even more following my suggestions; they have dropped that much within twelve months, and they have held that weight off for a long time.

THE FINISH of Dieting goes a step beyond Intuitive eating. Not merely does it solution why eating health- completely often appears so difficult, it empowers you with the desire and capability to do so. In the next pages, I talk about the technology and the solutions behind how exactly to rid yourself once and for all of the meals addictions sabotaging your wellbeing. I construct an easy-to-follow eating system you start with a fourteen-day group of easy-to-make, delicious meals that will steadily transform your food preferences, while concurrently recalibrating your palate. I guide your meal options through the first section of the program, so you don't need to think or be concerned in what you're eating-you can merely eat tasty dishes manufactured from fantastic health-assisting foods. In the next area of the programme, I flood the body with nutrition to heal and detoxify it, using very foods in an effort to promote wellness and longevity. By completing and sticking with the program, your BMI shall fall below 22.5 and stay there for the others you will ever have.

A diet can just be looked at successful if the meals you eat helps longevity and protect you against cardiovascular disease, stroke, dementia, and malignancy. This nutritarian diet design is the just dietary and nutritional system that guarantees dramatic excess weight reduction without calorie counting. Additionally, it is the just dietary and nutritional plan that explains how to drive back disease while simultaneously significantly increasing your lifespan. Your threat of a coronary attack and/or stroke will almost disappear, and your threat of tumour can plummet by a lot more than 90 per cent, while your daily life expectancy can boost by two decades. Incredible statements, yes, but that is a reality with substantial scientific support. I've observed such outcomes for a lot more than twenty-five years. Forget calorie consumption. The trick of living well is about micronutrients. Eating healthfully and consuming the proper assortment and quantity of nutrients outcomes in consistent, long-term health benefits. Getting healthful and maintaining well balanced, healthful weights are achieved just by concentrating on the dietary quality of your meal. Contrary to standard thinking, it isn't just how much you take in that determines your body weight; it's everything you eat.

Nutritional quality determines your mental, physical, and psychological health-from brain function and an elevated disease fighting capability to happiness and physical well-being. The primary criterion you should think about when choosing what things to eat is which foods are most favourable to your long-term survival. A diet plan style incorporating longevity- advertising foods enables you to try out all sorts of delicious quality recipes, which allows you to continue this new method of eating through the entire rest you will ever have. Any diet you adopt temporarily only results in short-term benefits because eventually your body and your weight change back to the diet you will remain in the long term. I want to repeat that again: Whatever you adopt temporarily just begets temporary outcomes, and fluctuating your body weight up and down isn't life- span favourable. People often view diet programs as a belief program, picking the one which is most closely aligned with their dietary philosophy or food preferences. They often criticize any system that conflicts with these choices. Real science, however, does not have any philosophy or predetermined agenda; it simply flows inexorably from the preponderance of the data. Are you a scientific thinker? Do you want to view reality and allow chips to fall with the data? Remember: Food choices are learned and may be changed.

We have cared for a lot more than 10 thousand people, the majority of whom set foot in my own office unhappy, sick, and overweight. That they had tried each and every dietary craze without achievement. After following my plan, they found out the superior health they always wanted and dropped the weight they always dreamed of losing. Even better, it was kept by them off. For the very first time in their lives, that they had a feeding on the style that didn't keep them starving or unsatisfied. Most of all, they were in a position to stop acquiring their medicines, which had become unneeded.

In the last three decades, I've reviewed a lot more than twenty thousand scientific tests on human nutrition. For this reason, I can state with certainty that is usually the place and today is the period to begin your wellbeing revival. I've seen the results of this plan doing his thing on a large number of people with a wide variety of diseases and health issues, from migraines and allergies to cardiovascular disease and diabetes. The end result is, it functions. Nutritional excellence may be the most effective way to discover long term healthy weight reduction, prevent and invert disease, and end a few of today's most chronic degenerative illnesses.

Your body is a self-therapeutic machine when you supply it with an optimal nutritional environment, and the information presented in this book is the quickest and most effective way to create that environment. In case you have high blood circulation pressure, high cholesterol, diabetes, cardiovascular disease, indigestion, headaches, asthma, exhaustion, body aches, or discomfort- or if you would like to avoid yourself from developing these chronic conditions-this may be the arrange for you. This fresh diet style can allow you in order to avoid angioplasty, bypass medical procedures, and other invasive methods. In the event that you aren't however ill, it could make sure you do not have heart episodes, strokes, or dementia in your old age. It can reduce and eventually get rid of your need for prescription drugs. In short, it can allow you to optimize your health and potentially save your life. And it could do all this while raising the enjoyment you get from meals. A lot of you have this publication because you would like to lose weight. I wish to assure you that you'll lose all of the weight that you would like, even if diet programs have failed you previously. This is usually the most reliable weight-loss plan ever, and the email address details are permanent, not temporary. Equally essential may be the protection from severe diseases in your own future that this plan gives. The most efficient healthcare is self-care. Medicines and doctors can't grant you superb health insurance and protect you from disease and suffering. Almost every doctor does know this. The dietary excellence I explain in the following can prevent and actually reverse most medical complications within three to half a year. That is a bold state, but the facts- supported by scientific research-display that lots of the tragedies we encounter in today's world are the consequence of nutritional folly. While weight reduction is important, it isn't our main objective. It is an enjoyable and regular by-product on the path to the principal goal: great health. First-class health is definitely marked by an exceedingly long and fairly disease-free lifespan, and countless research reveals that individuals with superior wellness are thin. By teaching you how exactly to achieve superior health, your ideal weight will normally follow. You will understand the physical cravings that trigger overeating, along with the psychological factors that will help you switch this pattern of usage. Applying the info in this reserve to your life can help you create new, healthy behaviours that may eventually become effortless. You will finally maintain control of your health destiny.

This plan will not include counting calories, measuring food portion sizes, or weighing. It doesn't depend on gimmicks or fads. You can end searching for that magic answer since there is no magic remedy. No reddish berry ketones. No green coffees. No purple tulip nectar or dark salt from the white cliffs of Dover. Actually, we almost always, later on, discover that the merchandise that gave us wish was simply hype and that searching for a magic pill causes harm. Whenever a supplement or medicine doesn't meet up with your nutritive requirements, it really is typically toxic and may enhance the damage the effect of a toxic diet. As we struggled with these issues, we started to explore a few of the popular literature that suggested a 180-level departure from dieting. It proposed a means of consuming that allowed for just about any and all meals choices, regardless of nutrition. Our preliminary reactions were extremely sceptical, if not down- correct rejecting. We reacted with self-righteous indignation. How could we, as nutritionists (authorized dietitians), trained to consider the connections between nourishment and health, sanction a means of eating that appeared to reject the foundation of our understanding and philosophy?

The struggle continued. Healthy eating plans did not help people maintain long-term weight control; the "nutritional waste strategy" was a dangerous choice. The suggestion to ignore nutrition and disregard the way the body seems in response to eating "whatever you want" discount rates the respect for one's body that comes combined with the gift of life. Finally, we resolved the conflict by developing the process of intuitive consumption. This book may be a bridge between its growing movement against diet and the medical community. While the anti-diet movement avoids dieting and blames body acceptance (thankfully), it often doesn't address health risks. How can you reconcile the problems of forbidden foods but still eat healthy, without dieting? We will let you know how in this post.

In case you are like most of our customers, you are tired of dieting but at the same time terrified of eating. Most of our customers feel uncomfortable within their bodies, but don't understand how to change. Intuitive eating provides a new way of eating that is ultimately hassling free and healthy for the brain and body. It really is an activity that frees the chains of the diet (which can only cause deprivation, rebellion and weight gain in extension). This means getting back again to your roots-trusting the body and its signals.

Intuitive eating cannot only change the relationship with food; it can change your daily life.

Intuitive Feeding on includes the principles of mindful eating; in addition, it has a broader philosophy, addressing the problems of cognitive distortions and psychological eating. It includes seeing realization as a central point in consumption, physical activity/movement in relation to feeling good, rejecting the mentality of the diet, using nutritional information without judging and respecting the body, regardless of how you feel about your shape. Intuitive nutrition is undoubtedly a dynamic procedure that integrates the tuning of the brain, body and meals. For those with feeding problems, conscious and intuitive feeding can help facilitate normal feeding.

Chapter 1:
Hitting the Diet Bottom

I just can't get on with another diet plan; you are my last resort." Sandra has been on a diet her entire existence and has understood that she could no longer support a single diet program. She had been with all of them, Atkins, Dukan, The Area, South Beach, grapefruit diet ... too many diets for the details. Sandra was a professional on a diet. Initially, the diet was fun, even stimulating. "Usually, I thought this diet will be different right now." So the routine would be reloaded with every fresh diet, every summer. But the lost weight would eventually be recovered as an undesirable tax bill.

Sandra had hit bottom in the diet plan. At this point, however, I was even more obsessed with meals and her body than ever. She felt silly. "I would have managed and controlled this in the past." What he did not understand was that the dietary procedure had been carried out. Dieting made her even more worried about meals. Diet had made enemy meals. The acquired diet made his experience guilty when he did not consume dietary foods (although she was not officially on a diet). Dieting experienced slowed her metabolism.

Sandra took years to understand that the diet does not work (yes, she knew the emerging idea that the diet does not work, but usually thought it would be different). Some experts and consumers recognize the premise that fast diets don't work: it is difficult for a country of people who are enthusiastic about their bodies to think that even a "practical diet" is often useless. Sandra has been hooked by the interpersonal mythology of the modern age group, the "great hope of diet", for most of her lifestyle since her first diet program at the age of fourteen.

At thirty, Sandra felt trapped: she still wanted to lose weight and was uncomfortable in her body. While Sandra couldn't bear the very thought of another diet plan, she didn't understand that the majority of her food problems were actually due to her dieting. Sandra was also discouraged and angry-"I understand everything about diets." Certainly, she could recite calorie consumption and fat grams, just like a walking dietary data source. This is the big warning of losing excess weight and avoiding it usually isn't a problem of understanding. If all we had to have a normal weight was to understand food and nutrition, most people in the United States would not be overweight. The information is easily available. (Take any women's magazine, and you will find abundant diet plans and comparisons with meals).

In addition, the more you try to follow the diet, the more you will fall (it certainly hurts to never succeed in case you have done the best). The best description due to this effect is distributed by John Foreyt, Ph.D., one of the leading professionals of diet psychology. He compared it to a Chinese puzzle (the hollow straw cylindrical puzzle, in which an index finger is placed on each end). The more you try to get out, the more pressure you will exert, the harder it will be to escape the puzzle. Instead, you find yourself locked up in a narrower place ... caught ... frustrated.

SYMPTOMS OF DIET PLAN BACKLASH

Diet backlash may be the cumulative side-effect of dieting-it could be short-term or chronic, depending on how long one has been dieting. It can only be one or more side effects. When Sandra got to any office, she already had the traditional symptoms of a violent reaction to the diet. Not only was she tired of following a diet, but she ate less food, but she also had problems losing weight during her new diet attempts. Additional symptoms include:

a. The simple contemplation of starting a diet causes desires and cravings for "sinful" and "fatty" foods, such as ice cream, chocolate, biscuits, etc.
b. When you quit a diet, go overeating and feel guilty. One research indicated that post- dieting binges happen in 49 per cent of most individuals who end a diet.

c. Have low self-esteem with meals. It's understandable that every diet program taught you never to trust the body or the food you dedicate. Although it may be the procedure for the diet that fails, failure continues to undermine its romantic relationship with food.

d. Since you don't deserve to consume because you're overweight.

e. Reduced duration of the diet. Living on a diet is getting shorter. (It could be indisputable that the Ultra Slim-Fast sales page is "Give us weekly ... and we ..."

f. Last dinner. All diet plans are preceded by foods that you presume not to eat anymore. Food consumption often increases during this period. It can happen with a meal or in a few days. The last supper seems to be the last step before the "nutritional cleansing", almost a farewell party. For a single customer, Marilyn, each meal seemed to be the last. I ate every meal until it filled up uncomfortable since I was terrified that I would never eat again. Once for all reasons! He was on a diet because the first grade exceeded two-thirds of his existence! He experienced provisional fasting intervals and a series of low-calorie diets. As for his body, the diets were just around the corner, so it's best to eat when you can. Any food for Marilyn was a relief from hunger.

g. Social abstinence. Since it is difficult to go on a diet and visit a party or go out for dinner, it is easier to refuse social invitations. At first, social avoidance of food may seem wiser for dieting reasons, but it becomes a big deal. There is often the concern of being able to maintain static control. It is not unusual for this meeting to be strengthened by "maintaining calorie intake or excess grams of fat for the party", which often means eating almost nothing. But by enough time the dieter finds the party, ravenous food cravings dominates and consuming feels very uncontrollable.

h. Sluggish metabolism. Each diet plan shows your body to adjust better to another purposeful starvation (another eating routine arrangement). The digestion backs off as the body utilizes each calorie successfully, as though it were the last. The more extreme the eating routine, the more it will push your body into the endurance condition that diminishes calories. Bolstering your digestion is like filling a fire. Expel the strong wood, and the fire diminishes. Essentially, to build the pace of digestion, we should eat a satisfactory measure of calories; generally, our life structures will redress and back off.

i. Use caffeine to endure the day. Espresso and diet drinks will, in general, be manhandled as a supervisory group to feel fiery while eating pretty much nothing.

j. Eating disorder. At long last, for a few, the rehashed diet is generally the foundation of a dietary problem (going from anorexia nervosa or bulimia to impulsive indulging).

Despite the fact that Sandra felt she could never again follow dieting, she was as yet engaged with the most recent wonder of the Supper. (We frequently meet him each time we see somebody just because.) Truth be told, she ate higher nourishment levels than expected and ate huge numbers of her preferred nourishments (he figured he could never observe these kinds of nourishment again). It seems as though you are arranging a long outing and planning additional garments. The straightforward thought of concentrating on her eating issues put her in the attitude of the pre-diet plan, something normal.

While Sandra essentially started to comprehend the worthlessness of the dieting, she should be slim had not changed, obviously a predicament. She clung to the appeal of honourable American want.

THE PARADOX OF DIETING

Inside our general public, the quest for slenderness (both for wellbeing and physical make-up) has wound up being the call to war of clearly all Americans. Eating an individual nibble of any nourishment that is high in fat or non-healthfully redeemable is generally deserving of a "blameworthy" expression by affiliation. You may be paroled, in any case, for "extraordinary conduct." Good conduct, inside our way of life, implies beginning a crisp eating routine or having incredible aims to abstain from food. Along these lines starts the hardship routine of dieting- the battle of the "bulge and indulge". Rice cakes for seven days, Häagen-Dazs the following.

"I feel remorseful essentially for enabling the staple worker to perceive what I purchase," said another client, who by chance had his trolley loaded with a natural product, vegetables, entire grains, pasta and a little 16 ounces of genuine dessert. It seems as though we were in a state of utilization of the Food Law coordinated by the nourishment mafia. Furthermore, there consistently is by all accounts dieting you can't refuse. Embellishment? No. We are sensible for this discernment.

A report distributed in 1993 in Eating Disorders-The Journal of Treatment and Avoidance found that somewhere in the range of 1973 and 1991, notices for dietary guides (diet nourishments, nourishment decrease helps, and diet programs) expanded practically direct. The analysts likewise referenced that there is absolutely a parallel model at the beginning of utilization issue. It is speculated that the weight of the push on the dietary arrangement (through publicizing spots) for the most part importantly affects the pattern of buyer unsettling influence.

The dieting pressure plan is powered past TV ads. Magazine articles and film content add to the weight of being thin. Fragile cigarette announcements additionally go for the heaviness of the Achilles female heel with titles like Ultra Thin 100, Virginia Slims, and so forth. A Kent cigarette, "Thin Lights", explicitly portrays this push on ladies' physical issues. Your promotion is like that of an industrialist for a decrease in normal weight contrasted with a cigarette, featuring lean depictions: "long", "slight", "light". Obviously, the examples in cigarette ads are especially unpretentious. Obviously, the inside for disease control (CDC) traits and expansion in ladies' smoking to their need to be more slender. Tragically, we have heard ladies ponder in our workplaces who have likewise viewed as smoking again as a guide to getting more fit.

Be that as it may, weight reduction isn't only a worry of ladies (albeit clearly there is extra weight on ladies). The multiplication of business contributions of light lager has planted the seed of body mindfulness in men's considerations; in addition, a fit stomach is desirable over one of brew. It is no occurrence that we have seen the dispatch of magazines focused on men, for example, Males Fitness and Female's Health. While the quest for slenderness has crossed the sexual orientation boundary, we have sadly brought forth the original of weight onlookers — an upsetting pattern towards new dieting influences the wellness of American youngsters. Stunning exploration has shown that school-age kids are fixating on their weight-an impression of a nation eager about dieting and overabundance weight. The nation over, six-year-olds are getting thinner, scared of putting on weight, and being continuously treated for utilization issue that compromises their wellbeing and development protection. Social strain to shed pounds has bombed in kids. Not exclusively can eating less junk food work; it is generally the principle issue. Albeit many may follow dieting as a push to lose abundance weight or for wellbeing reasons, the conundrum is clearly that it could cause more damage. This is the thing that our nation must show to the eating routine:

a. Obesity is greater than any time in recent memory in grown-ups and youngsters.
b. Dietary problems are on the ascent.
c. Child weight issues have multiplied in the previous ten years.
d. Despite the way that there are still more without fat and dietary nourishments than previously, just about 66% of grown-ups are hefty or fat.
e. More than one thousand 200 and a lot of fat has just been liposuction from 1982 to 1992. (And as of late accessible review indicated that once a year after a liposuction procedure, fat returned, yet in another area of the body).
f. Diet builds the possibility to increase significantly a greater number of pounds than you have lost!

DIETING INTAKE CANNOT BATTLE BIOLOGY
Diet is a kind of transient yearning. Accordingly, when you are given a principal chance to eat truly, you experience so firmly that you feel wild, an edgy demonstration. With respect to natural yearning, all expectations to design the eating routine and the need to get in shape are temporary and incomprehensibly superfluous. In those concise minutes, we become simply like the voracious man-expending plant in the film Little Store of Horrors, testing to eat-"Feed me, feed me."

While outrageous eating may appear to be crazy and unnatural, it is really a standard reaction to yearning and diet. Notwithstanding, it can frequently be viewed as that eating after the dieting doesn't have "determination" or imperfection in character. Be that as it may, in translating the post-dietary nourishment plan accordingly, it gradually disintegrates fearlessness with nourishment, diet after eating routine. Each infringement of the eating routine arrangement, each nourishment situation that appears to be wild establishes the frameworks for the "diet plan mindset", step by step and diet by diet. The evidently daring arrangement invest more energy following time-transforms into as dumbfounding as the Chinese finger confound. You can't fight science. At the point when your body starves, it should be bolstered. In any case, frequently a weight watcher gripes: "Just on the off chance that I experience determination." Clearly, this isn't just a self-control issue. (In spite of the fact that the splendid tribute from fat misfortune treatment focuses support this lost blame in determination.) When you are not encouraged, you will get fixated on nourishment, regardless of whether on a purposeful eating routine or craving.

You can't count calories, yet eat cautiously for the sake of wellbeing. This is by all accounts the politically right term for "diet" during the 90s. Be that as it may, in any event, for some, it's a similar issue with dinners, with similar side effects. Keeping away from overabundance fats or sugars, whatever occurs, and subsisting on basically sans fat or starch-free nourishments is basically an eating routine and frequently brings about a lacking eating routine. There are numerous kinds of diets and different sorts of diets. We will investigate your dietary character and meet the Intuitive Eater in the following part.

DIET INCREASES YOUR RISK OF GETTING MORE WEIGHT!
On the off chance that dietary applications were to withstand a similar control as medications, open utilization probably won't be permitted. Envision, for instance, taking asthma to medicate, which improves relaxing for half a month; however, over the long haul; it exacerbates the lungs and relaxing. Will I truly follow an eating routine (a great supposed "reasonable eating routine"), in the event that I realized I could make you put on weight?

Here is a couple of calming research demonstrating that eating less junk food advances weight gain:

a. A gathering of UCLA specialists inspected thirty-one long haul investigated on eating less junk food and figured slimming down is a consistent indicator of overabundance weight gain-up to 66% of the individuals recovered more abundance weight than they dropped (Mann et al., 2007).
b. Research on almost seventeen thousand kids between the ages of nine and fourteen finished up: "... in the long haul, the weight-controlling eating routine isn't just ineffectual, yet could advance weight gain" (Field et al. 2003).
c. People on a high school diet had twice the same number of odds of being overweight than adolescents on dieting regarding a multiyear review. Specifically, toward the start of the examination, individuals on an eating routine don't gauge significantly more than their companions who don't follow dieting. This is a significant detail, provided that individuals on dieting weigh much more, it could be a component of perplexity (which would suggest extra factors, as opposed to counting calories, for example, genetics).

Epic research on more than 2,000 units of twins from Finland, matured 16 to 25 years matured indicated that consuming fewer calories itself, free of hereditary qualities, is impressively connected with quickened fat addition and expanded danger of getting stout (Pietilaineet et al. 2011). Dietary twins, who experienced a solitary purposeful health improvement plan, were just about a few times bound to be overweight than their non-dietary twin partner. Likewise, the plausibility of unreasonable overweight improved in a portion subordinate way with every dietary occasion.

Studies aside: what did your dietary experiences show you? Numerous people and individuals in the lab state their first dieting plan was straightforward: the pounds basically liquefied away. Yet, that first dietary experience could be the temptation trap, which starts the vain quest for weight decrease through eating routine. We state pointless on the grounds that our bodies are amazingly wise and designed for endurance.

Organically, your body experiences the dieting process predominantly in light of the fact that it is a sort of starvation. Your cells don't comprehend you are intentionally limiting your dinner admission. The body shifts into base endurance mode-digestion diminish, and nourishment needing heighten. What's more, with each diet plan, your body learns and adjusts, which prompts weight gain in expansion. Therefore, many people feel simply like they absolutely are a disappointment; however, it truly is eating less junk food which has bombed them.

Chapter 2:
What Type of Eater Are You?

You can continue on a diet and not know! There are many types of eating styles that are actually unconscious types of dieting. Quite a few people have said these were not really on a diet plan- but upon nearer inspection of what and how they consume, they were dieting still!

A good example here's. Ted arrived because he wished to lose excess weight. He said that in his fifty years of life, he had previously only been on four serious diet programs. In examining the titles of publications at work (compulsory overeating texts, consumption of books on ailments, etc.), he said: "You use many serious complications in the diet ... well, I'm not just one of those. Obviously, Ted did not consider himself a dietician, who ate simply with care, but showed that it was an unconscious diet.

Although Ted had not followed an active diet, he was eating at a level where he had almost passed out in the afternoon. The reason: he had been unhappy with his weight! In the morning I chose an intense bicycle trip down a hill, for only an hour. I would go back and have breakfast for a bit. Lunch was usually a salad with iced tea (although it seems healthy, it is too low in carbohydrates). At dinner time, your body will scream for meals. Ted not only had a severe calorie deficit, but he also lacked carbohydrates. Nights become a food party! Ted had the idea that it was previously a "food volume" problem with a solid sweet tooth. The truth is that previously he had an unconscious mentality in the diet that biologically triggered his night diet and his pleasant tooth.

Even Alicia hadn't been on a conscious diet. She never came to lose pounds, but because she wanted to increase her vitality. During the initial program, it became clear that he had problems with food. So they asked him if he had done many diets. She seemed amazed. "How did you know I did billions of diets?" While Alicia claimed to be comfortable with her current fat, she was still at war with food; she did not trust herself with meals. It turns out that Alicia has been on a diet since she was a child. Although he hadn't officially followed a diet, he maintained (and expanded) a couple of dietary guidelines with each diet plan that almost paralyzed her ability to eat normally. We observe this at all times, the hangover from dieting: avoiding certain foods no matter what, feeling uncontrollable as soon as a "sinful" meals are eaten, sense guilty when self-imposed food guidelines are broken (such as for example "Thou shalt not really eat previous to 6 P.M."), and so forth.

The unconscious diet usually occurs in the type of meticulous eating habits. There can be an excellent line between feeding on for health insurance and dieting. Notice how actually the frozen diet plan foods such as for example, Lean Cuisine and Excess weight Watchers are placing their focus on health instead of a diet. As long as you participate in some form of the diet, the recipient will eliminate food and body concerns. Whether you are a conscious or unconscious person, the results of the medial side are similar, the diet again, the effect of the eyelashes. It seems like a period in which one eats cautiously, "blowing" it and spending penance with an increase in diet or extremely cautious consumption. In this chapter, we will explore the many diet/nutrition styles to help see what your position is now. Later, you will meet the Intuitive Eater and the intuitive style of food, and the perfect solution is to live without diet programs.

THE EATING PERSONALITIES

To help you clarify your food design style (or diet), we have identified the following key types of eaters that feature distinctive food patterns: the careful eater, the one that makes a professional diet and the eater unconscious. These consuming personalities are exhibited even if they are not officially on a diet. It is possible to have significantly more than one consuming personality, although we find that there is commonly a dominant trait. The chances of your life can also influence or change your personality to eat. For example, a client, a tax attorney, was usually a careful eater, but during the fiscal period of the year, it became the chaotic unconscious eater.

It is possible that it occasionally possesses the intake characteristics described below in the three nuclei that feed on personality. Note this, and if your feed exists in one of these domains most of the time, it's a problem.

Review each character you eat and see which one best reflects your style. By understanding what your position is now, it will be easier to find out how to become an intuitive eater. For example, you may find that you have already been involved in a type of diet and have not even recognized it. Or you can discover features that, without knowing it, work against you.

THE CAREFUL EATER
Cautious consumers are those who tend to be attentive to the food they put into their bodies. Ted was a good example of a careful eater (per day). At the top, accurate eaters look like "ideal" eaters. They are highly aware of nutrition. Externally, they seem oriented towards health and fitness (noble characteristics admired and strengthened in our society).

Style
There is a selection of eating behaviours exhibited by Careful Eater. In an intense moment, Cautious Eater can be distressed for every bite of food allowed in the body. Shopping trips are spent looking at meal labels. Eating out can indicate interrogating the waiter what's in the meals, how maybe the meals prepared-and obtaining assurances that the meals are prepared particularly to the Cautious Eater's liking (not often one speck of essential oil or other excess fat used). What's incorrect with this? Aren't label reading and assertive cafe ordering in the medical interests of some individuals? Of program! However, the difference could be the vigilante force and the ability to forget any defect related to the choice of consumption. Attentive eaters tend to consume less than

normal and control the amount of food consumed. The attentive eater can spend most of his waking hours planning another meal or snack, often worried about eating. Since Careful Eater is not officially on a diet, your brain punishes all the "harmful", fatty or sugary foods you eat. The Careful Eater can travel the fine line between sincerely thinking about health and eating carefully with respect to body image.

Sometimes, Careful Eater is driven by periods or events. For example, some careful eaters are meticulous during weekdays, to make sure they get their "ideal of consumption" to "show off" on the weekends or for the next party. But on weekends they happen 104 times a year: waste can be counterproductive with unwanted weight gain. Consequently, it is not uncommon for a cautious eater to think about starting a diet.

The Problem
There's nothing incorrect with being thinking about the well-being of the body. However, the problem occurs when diligent consumption (almost in contact with the militant) affects a healthy relationship with food and negatively affects the body. Prudent eaters, on closer inspection, resemble a delicate diet style. They can't be on a diet; however, they look into every food scenario.

THE PROFESSIONAL DIETER
People on a professional diet are easier to identify; they are on a perpetual diet. In general, they tried the latest commercial diet, the diet book or the trick to lose weight. Sometimes, the diet is performed in the form of fasting or "reduction". Professional Dieters understand a whole lot about portions of foods, calories, and "dieting methods," yet the cause they are usually on another diet plan is that the initial one never worked. Today, Professional Dieter can be amply trained in counting carbohydrate grams.

Style
People on a professional diet also have accurate food traits. The difference, however, is that people on a diet chronically, guiding the choice of meals to lose weight, not necessarily for

health. When the dieter is not officially on a diet, he generally thinks about the next diet that can be started. He often wakes up wishing this is a good day, the fresh start. While people on a professional diet have a lot of knowledge of diets, they don't serve them well. It is not uncommon to allow them to eat compulsively or participate in the consumption of the Last Supper as soon as a prohibited meal is eaten. This is because people on a chronic diet really believe that they will no longer eat this food; tomorrow I'm on a diet, tomorrow they start again with a clean slate. Better eat right now; it's the last opportunity. And in addition, the Professional Dieter gets discouraged at the futility of the vicious routine. Diet, lose weight, put on weight, intermittent binges, and back again to dieting.

The Problem

It's very difficult to live in this manner. The Yo-Yo diet helps make losing excess weight more difficult as well as eating healthy. Chronic lack of food usually causes overeating or periodic feeding. For some diet professionals, the frustration of losing weight intensifies so much that they can try laxatives, diuretics and weight loss supplements. And trigger that these "dietary aids" generally don't work, they could try extreme methods like chronic restriction, in the type of anorexia nervosa or bleeding (like nausea after a binge), in the type of bulimia. While anorexia and bulimia are multifactorial and have their roots in psychological problems, a growing body of research suggests that chronic diet is usually a common step towards an eating disorder. One study specifically found that when enough dieters reach the age of fifteen, they are eight times more likely to have problems with an eating disorder than people who don't go on a diet.

THE UNCONSCIOUS EATER
The Unconscious Eater is often engaged in a paired diet, which consists of eating and simultaneously doing another activity, such as watching television and eating, or eating and reading. Due to the subtleties and insufficient awareness, it can become problematic for a person to recognize this eating character. There are numerous subtypes of unconscious eaters.

THE CHAOTIC UNCONSCIOUS EATER
Live a life that is too often programmed, too busy, too many things you can do. The chaotic, consuming design is haphazard; whatever's obtainable will end up being grabbed-vending machine fare, junk food, it'll all perform. Food and diet tend to be vital to this person-just not really in the critical instant of the chaos. Chaotic eaters tend to be so busy putting out fires that have difficulty identifying biological cravings for food until it is fiercely voracious. And in addition, the chaotic eater will go extended periods of time without eating.

THE REFUSE-NOT UNCONSCIOUS EATER
They are vulnerable to the simple existence of food, regardless of whether they are hungry or full. The jars of sweets, the meals at the meetings, the food sitting on the kitchen counter, probably none of them will be overcome. However, most of the time, it is fair; consumers who do not refuse to consume are not aware of what they are consuming or how much they consume. For example, the Reject-Not Eater can actually pick up some candy on the way to the bathroom without being aware of it. Social outings that revolve around meals such as cocktails and festive buffets are particularly difficult for Refuse-Not Eater.

THE WASTE-NOT UNCONSCIOUS EATER
Evaluate meals in dollars. His / her eating travel is frequently influenced by getting just as much as they are able to your money can buy. Waste-Not Eater is particularly inclined to completely clean the plate (and also that of others). It is not unusual for a waste eater not to actually consume the leftovers of children or spouse.

THE UNCONSCIOUS EMOTIONAL EATER
They use food to manage emotions, especially unpleasant feelings such as stress, anger and loneliness. While Emotional Eaters look at their consuming as the problem, it's often a sign of a deeper concern. Consuming behaviours of the Emotional Eater can range between grabbing a bag of chips on stressful occasions to chronic compulsive binges of huge quantities of food.

The problem

Unconscious power, in its many forms, usually be a problem if it translates into persistent excessive consumption (which can simply occur if you are eating instead of being very alert). Remember that somewhere between the first and last bite of meals is where the awareness period actually occurs. Like in "Oh, it's all over!"

For example, have you ever bought a large package of candy in the movies and started consuming it, and then you find that your fingertips suddenly scratch themselves under the empty container? This is a simple type of unconscious feeding. But unconscious nutrition can also exist at an extreme level, in a relatively altered feeding condition. In this case, the individual is not attentive to what is consumed, why he has started eating, or how he knows about the taste of the food. That is zoning out with meals.

WHEN YOUR EATING PERSONALITY WORKS AGAINST YOU
Finally, the food varieties of Careful Eater, Professional Dieter and Unconscious Eater become an inefficient feeding method, even if at the top they seem to be fine. The perfect solution is for the discouraged consumer: try more with a fresh diet! At first, the new diet seems stimulating and hopeful, but in the end, the family pounds return. The diet becomes more demanding, and even if you resume your basal consumption personality, you may feel more unpleasant than before. It is because internal dietary guidelines are strengthened with each diet plan. These meal rules often perpetuate the guilt emotions of consumption, even when you are not officially on a diet. Furthermore, the biological ramifications of the diet make it increasingly difficult to have a normal romantic relationship with meals. The Intuitive Eater character, however, can be an exception. It's the only feeding design that doesn't work against you and will help you end chronic diets and yo-yo weight fluctuations.

INTUITIVE EATER INTRODUCTION
Intuitive eaters march with their signs of internal hunger and eat regardless of what they choose without feeling guilty or an

ethical dilemma. The intuitive eater can be an independent eater. However, it is increasingly difficult to become an unaltered eater in today's health-conscious society considering the bombardment of communications on food, food and weight by advertisers, the press and medical researchers. When we explained the basic feeding characteristics of Intuitive Eater to its customers, it is surprising how often we will hear the answer: "This is how my partner eats." This or how my boyfriend eats. "When we ask what the person's weight and romantic relationship is with food, the answer is: "No problem!" Consider small children. Intuitive, natural eaters will be practically free of social messages about meals and body image. Toddlers possess innate wisdom of meals, in the event that you don't hinder it. They don't eat predicated on dieting guidelines or health, yet study after research shows that if you allow a toddler consumes spontaneously; he'll eat what he requirements when given free usage of food. (This is most likely the toughest point for a concerned mother or father to do- to release and trust that children have an innate capability to eat!)

This is true even when food for food, food for little tykes is apparently a father's nightmare. Experts found that calorie intake was highly variable in confirmed foods; However, it has been balanced over time. However, many parents assume that their children cannot properly regulate their diet. As a result, parents often adopt coercive strategies in an attempt to ensure that the child eats a nutritionally sufficient diet. But a previous study by Birch and his colleagues indicates that these control strategies are countered. In addition, Birch notes that "parents' attempts to regulate their children's feeding have been reported more regularly by obese adults than by normal-weight adults." Likewise, Duke University psychologist Philip Costanzo, PhD found that unwanted weight in school-age children was closely related to the level at which parents sought to limit their children's food. Actually, well-meaning parents hinder Intuitive Eating. Whenever a mother or father attempts to overrule a child's organic eating cues, the nagging problem gets worse, not better. A parent, who feeds a kid every time a hunger signal is heard and who stops feeding when the infant demonstrates he's had enough, may play a robust role in the original development of Intuitive Feeding on. Indeed, the innovative role of the therapist and dietician offered by Ellyn Satter has shown that, in the event that the parents of obese children cool down and allow them to consume without the pressure of their parents, the children will ultimately eat much less. Why? The child begins to listen and understand his internal signs of hunger and satiety. The child also knows that he will use food. According to Satter, "children deprived of food so that they can lose weight, worry about food, fear they don't have enough to eat and are susceptible to overeating if they get the chance." We have found that this is accurate for dieters too. Limited to adults, the intuitive drinking process has been buried over a long period, often years and years. Instead of relaxing a father's pressure, this decrease in pressure should be the result of inside and against the myth of society about dieting and distorted body worship. Fortunately, we all have the natural ability to eat intuitively; It has simply been suppressed, especially with the diet. This book specializes in showing you exactly how to wake the intuitive eater in you.

HOW YOUR INTUITIVE EATER GETS BURIED
As toddlers get yourself a little older, the mixed messages start to creep in-from the early influences of the Saturday morning food commercial, to the well-meaning mother or father who coaxes his kid to "Clean your plate." The assault won't stop if you're a kid. There are many external forces that impact our eating, that may include additionally bury Intuitive Eating.

DIETING
You have already seen the damage from a chronic diet, which includes, among others:

    a. Increase in excessive consumption
    b. Decreased metabolic rate.
    c. Greater concern about meals.
    d. Increase the emotions of deprivation.
    e. A greater sense of failure
    f. Reduced feeling of willpower.

This only serves to erode your confidence in food and prompts you to rely on external sources to guide your diet (one diet, one diet and enough time of the day, food rules, etc.). The more you head to external resources to "judge" if your consuming is in balance, the additional removed you feel from Intuitive Eating. Intuitive Eating depends on your inner cues and signals.

EAT HEALTHY MESSAGES OR DIE

Messages about healthy eating are everywhere, from nonprofit healthcare organizations to food companies promoting the medical benefits of their unique item. The inherent message? Everything you consume can improve your wellbeing. Conversely, take one incorrect move (bite), and you're one step nearer to the grave. Is usually this an exaggeration? No. For example, a 1994 press release published by the Harvard College of Public Health mentioned that the consumption of trans-fatty acids (inside margarine) could cause thirty thousand deaths each year in the United States due to cardiovascular disease. That sort of message can easily keep you feeling guilty for consuming the "incorrect" kind of meals and feeling puzzled in what you should eat.

Magazines and newspapers have also significantly increased their protection of food and well-being. A food publisher, Joe Crea, of an important metropolitan newspaper, the Orange County Register (California), said that in a period of six to 12 months (1987-1993) his stories about food multiplied by five. Of nearly eight hundred food stories, two hundred had been linked to health problems. Although there is absolutely no doubt that everything you eat can affect your health, exponential coverage of the press has been offered as a channel for the development of food paranoia in the purchaser, particularly in the diet. Joe Crea agrees: "Open the newspaper, visit a good story about cheesecake and, at the same time, another piece on how eating too much will make you gain weight. Place the incompatible player.

Are we saying you should ignore the virtues of healthy intake? Of course not. However, if you have a diet adapted to your diet, the burst of "healthy eating" messages can make you feel more guilty about the foods you choose to eat. Obesity and Wellness reported a study of 2,075 adults in Florida that revealed that 45% of adults felt guilty after eating the foods they liked. (Remember that this study was carried out to reflect common American demographics. These "guilt-by- eating" figures would probably be higher if performed on dieters.)

Women could be particularly guilty. A Gallup poll by the American Dietetic Association showed that women feel more guilty than men for the foods they eat (44 per cent versus 28 per cent). Could this be because females diet more often than men? Or because ladies are usually the prospective of health communications and food advertisements (consider the number of women's magazines). Women will be primarily responsible for decisions relating to family health care and will often also be responsible for food and nutritional problems; They serve as the main objective.

We have found that establishing a healthy diet or diet as a short priority in the intuitive feeding process is counterproductive. We initially ignore nutrition, as it interferes with the relearn process of an intuitive eater. Nutrition heresy? No. Food can be respected and honoured. It simply cannot be the first priority when you've been on a diet for a lifetime. Or consider it this way; in case you have focused all your attention on the diet, does it help you? The many nutritious diet programs (absolute) may become embraced as another type of diet.

Chapter 3:
Intuitive Eating Standards:
Summary

Just once he vows to dispose of the diet and supplant it with an activity focused on intuitive nourishing, is he considering escaping jail from abundance weight variances and food fixations? In this part, we will present the fundamental ideas of intuitive sustaining: a preview of every idea, with an examination study or two. The most significant aftereffect of every customer referenced was that of acquiring a sound association with dinners and their bodies. By following ten intuitive eating ideas, you will standardize your sentimental association with food. A focus on weight reduction must be set aside for later. On the off chance that your present pounds offer came about because of getting withdrawn together with your inward insight about eating, and subsequently, of tuning back into this intelligence, weight reduction happens, along these lines be it. Assuming, by the by, you are as of now keeping your set point fat through the action of limiting, overeating, confining, and so forth, at that point, it truly is particularly essential that you put weight to decrease on the storage compartment burner.

GUIDELINE ONE:

DECLINES THE MENTALITY OF THE DIETARY PLAN
Dispense with diet books and magazine articles that give you the bogus any desire for getting more fit rapidly, effectively and for all time. Feel furious about the falsehoods that made you sense that you had flopped each time a new diet quit working and you recovered all your weight. On the off chance that you enable a little want to demand that a crisp and better diet might be hiding close by, it will keep you from abstaining from rediscovering the intuitive diet.

For quite a while, we have sought after one diet plan for another, enabling the most stylish trend to direct what, how much, and when to eat. This inflexible way of life of limitation and hardship can bring about a dangerous association with food. The initial step on the intuitive sustenance scale is, for the most part, to depend on your impulses with respect to food decisions.

GUIDELINE TWO:

RESPECT YOUR HUNGER
Keep your body organically encouraged with adequate vitality and sugars. Else you can bring about base travel to indulge. When you reach the top appetite, all aims of moderate, conscious eating are passing and unessential. Seeing how to respect this first organic sign units the phase for revamping trust with yourself and dinners.

While most diets need you to object to a growling stomach, intuitive nutrition renews your body's signals. You'll make sense of how to be increasingly aware of your food yearnings and how precisely to react appropriately to it before you feel hungry. Attempt this in the home: Before each dinner, rate your level of yearning, record a couple of internal signals that you saw, and enough time of day. Do this for week by week, and you'll are more in order together with your hunger, and furthermore which foods convey dependable vitality and the ones that are quickly catching fire and convey short-lived satiety.

GUIDELINE THREE:

MAKE PEACE WITH FOOD
Call a détente; quit the food battle! Give unconditional approval to food. In the event that you illuminate yourself that you can't or shouldn't have a particular food, it can bring about serious feelings of hardship that incorporate with wild longings and, regularly, gorging. At the point when you at last "give up" to your illegal foods, eating will be acquainted with such force, it, for the most part, results in Last Supper overeating and

overpowering blame. Intuitive eating solicits that you forsake the idea from awful and the great food. That system energizes an unsafe 'win big or bust by any stretch of the imagination' attitude that may bring about longings for 'taboo' foods, joined by gorging and a rush of self-hatred and disgrace. Intuitive eating advances the hypothesis that food ought to be viewed as an actual existence upgrading experience.

GUIDELINE FOUR:

CHALLENGE THE MEALS POLICE
Shout a boisterous "basically no" to contemplations in your mind that proclaim you're "extraordinary" for eating under one thousand calories or "horrendous" in light of the fact that you ate a touch of chocolate cake. THE MEALS LAW AUTHORIZATIONS POLICE, the nonsensical rules that dieting has created. The police headquarters is certainly housed somewhere down in your mind, and its own amplifier yells ominous points, sad expressions, and blame inciting arraignments. Pursuing the suppers Police aside is a significant advance in time for Intuitive Eating. An escalated mental housekeeping and reframing disposition toward suppers are pivotal. Watch any food law authorization considerations you may have, such as "I was poor today" or "I shouldn't eat that." Resist the possibility that your food alternatives characterize it and the value it brings to the world. Pay special mind to people who might be deliberately or unwittingly showing a food police mindset, at that point talk about your intuitive eating way of thinking with them and have them to help you by hushing up about their terrible remarks.

GUIDELINE FIVE:

FEEL YOUR FULLNESS
Tune in for the body flags that let you realize that you are not any hungrier. Pay heed to the signs that show that you're effectively full. Interruption in the focal point of suppers or nibble and have yourself the manner in which the food tastes, and what your present completion level is.

The other side of regarding your appetite is to regard when you're full. Since diet programs limit what, when, and exactly the amount you expend, it's easy to get detached from the internal signs that transmission satiety. At the point when you practice intuitive expending you take up a feast with a lesser degree of food yearnings and in a mentality which enables you to turn out to be increasingly fragile to prompts that you're full. In addition, you comprehend that you could refuel at whatever point you're ravenous once more, and you won't encounter constrained to clean your plate totally. Evaluate this at home: Make utilization of a satiety scale all through suppers to prepare your brain to address signs of satiety. Record perceptions of how you are feeling and all that you ate. This can help decide when to leave the fork and let the dinners actually feel supported and empowered.

GUIDELINE SIX:

REVEAL THE SATISFACTION FACTOR
JAPAN has the knowledge to keep joy as you of their objectives of sound living. Inside our anger to be thin and sound, we regularly ignore likely the essential presents of presence the happiness and fulfilment, which can be inside the eating experience. At the point when you take in what you need, in a domain that is welcoming, the fulfilment you infer is incredible power in helping you are feeling fulfilled and content. By giving this experience to yourself, you will see that it takes essentially less food to pick; you've had "enough."

Intuitive eating urges you to perceive foods that really cause you to feel great all through supper, yet a short time later, as well. You will find yourself floating towards and time for the foods that produce you feel your absolute best. Besides to relishing suppers and eating groceries that taste extraordinary and make you feel incredible, you can connect the entirety of your faculties: slow down, acknowledge what kind of food looks, regard how it achieved your plate, inhale every one of the fragrances, and eat inside a domain that appears to be acceptable expedite the plants and candles-and with people who light you up.

GUIDELINE SEVEN:

ADAPT TOGETHER TO YOUR EMOTIONS WITHOUT NEEDING FOOD

Discover approaches to solace and simplicity, sustain, occupy, and illuminate your passionate worries without utilizing food. Stress, depression, weariness, and outrage are sentiments a large portion of us experience all through presence. Everyone has its trigger, and every offer its own conciliation. Suppers won't fix these sentiments. It could comfort for the present moment, divert from the distress, or really numb you directly into a food aftereffect. However, food won't solve the problem. In the event that anything, eating for an enthusiastic yearning is just going to make you feel more awful after some time. You'll, in the end, need to adapt to the wellspring of the feeling, alongside the distress of overeating.

Indeed, food could be encouraging, yet that delight just keeps going insofar as the food. A short time later, anything that was eating you stays, covered under food, perhaps now offered with a piece of blame and disgrace. Intuitive eating urges you to perceive whether you're sense on edge, exhausted, desolate, tragic, or irate and look for a veritable arrangement. Get a walk, call a dear companion, practice reflection or yoga, get a remedial back rub, read a composed book, or make in a diary. You'll comprehend you're reacting appropriately when the reaction empowers you to feel good, not more terrible.

GUIDELINE EIGHT:

RESPECT YOUR BODY

Acknowledge your hereditary outline. Just for the most part in light of the fact that an individual with a footwear size of eight wouldn't ordinarily foresee reasonably to crush directly into a size six, it truly is correspondingly useless (and horrendous) to have a comparable desire regarding the matter of body size. Regard the body, so you can encounter better about who you are. It's difficult to dismiss the dietary plan attitude in the event that you are ridiculous and excessively pivotal of the body shape.

Our varieties are our superpowers, but we live in a world that idealizes a cut body type. The possibility that individuals can profoundly change our life structures is typically unreasonable and ridiculous. Intuitive eating troubles you to grasp your hereditary plan set handy expectations, and praise your uniqueness. Evaluate this in the home: Anytime you catch yourself contrasting the body with someone else's, react as you'll if a buddy said something practically identical regarding themselves.

GUIDELINE NINE:

EXERCISE-FEEL THE DIFFERENCE
Disregard activist exercise. Just get dynamic and experience the distinction. Move your concentrate to how it appears to go your body, as opposed to the fat consuming limit impact of the activity. On the off chance that you focus on how you are feeling from working out, such as empowered, it could have the effect between turning up for an energetic morning hour's walk and striking the rest caution. If when you stirred, your solitary target is to lose abundance weight, rarely do you get an inspiring component at that time of period.

People who practice intuitive benefiting from appreciating practice since it gives them vitality improves their inclination, advances self-adequacy, and makes them experience solid, adaptable, and dexterous. Preparing isn't about which movement will consume off the most calories, however rather about which action might be the best time and stimulating. It's another exemplary instance of the manner in which the fulfilment factor could make propensities stick. The exercise you appreciate is an exercise that you're bound to do it once more, creating the force that drives feasible, long haul bliss.

GUIDELINE TEN:

RESPECT YOUR HEALTHY AND SOFT FOOD
Choose foods that respect your prosperity and taste buds while making you feel better. Comprehend that you don't have to eat a perfect diet to be invigorating. You won't all of a sudden get

yourself a supplement lack, or put on weight in one bite, one food, or one day of eating. It's what you normally eat after some time that issues. Progress, not so much flawlessness, is what makes a difference.

Recognizing how your prosperity impacts the wealth, you will ever have shallow known purposes behind health objectives and grounds your thought processes in what is important: your individual qualities. Getting the point of view on why health is significant can assist you with the understanding that no supper or chomp could represent the moment of truth your self-esteem. Adjust your prosperity to your aspirations, and you will be significantly progressively inspired to develop rehearses that help your day by day life objectives.

AN ACTIVITY WITH GREAT REWARDS
Numerous people have been disappointed with their association with food and their bodies. Many experienced endeavoured either formal or casual dieting and had encountered disappointment and gloom. By learning the ideas of Intuitive Consuming and putting them to work, many will find an extending of the evaluation of life and quality about eating. You can go as well!

Chapter 3:
Arousing the Intuitive Eater: Stages

The journey to Intuitive Eating is like going for a cross-district climbing trip. Before you really tie without anyone else climbing boots, you'd have to recognize what's in store all through your outing. While a road map is viable, it doesn't disclose what you'll be enough prepared, such as trail conditions, atmosphere, special touring detects, the kind of garments to put on, etc. The goal of this part is, for the most part, to help you comprehend what to envision all through your outing to Intuitive Eating.

Regardless of whether it's strolling or relearning an unmistakably all the more fulfilling eating plan, you will continue through numerous phases in transit. The amount of time that you should remain static in a specific stage is certainly a factor and amazingly individualized. For example, crossing new climbing trails relies on how physically fit you are, the way you adapt to worry with a new path, exactly how much time you have to climb, and the choice of climbing trails. In like manner, your adventure back again to Intuitive Eating relies on how protracted you've been dieting, how emphatically settled in your everyday diet believing is the means by which long you've been utilizing suppers to deal with life, that you are so arranged to confide in yourself, and that you are so prepared to put weight decrease on the storage compartment burner and see how to turn into an Intuitive Eater the essential objective.

Now and again, you'll move in reverse and advances among the stages. In the event that you recognize that is an ordinary segment of the procedure, it can assist you with continuing without inclination that you will fall away from the faith or not so much gaining ground.

Think about this circumstance: You are on a mobile path and experience a fork in the road that is difficult to unravel together with your path map. Do you go legitimately to one side or left? You consider for quite a while and pick to go remaining. While strolling, you place something you've in no way, shape or form seen previously, a sparkling green caterpillar shimmying up a purple bloom. A couple of activities ahead, you find a novel fowl. In any case, a couple of strategies past these wonders of character are a huge rock flagging that you locate an inappropriate course. You pivot, return to the fork, and think about the other course. Was this temporary re-routing an exercise in futility?

No! So also, in connection to Intuitive Eating, you will require numerous turns and test out new contemplations and practices. You may locate that subsequent to creating recognizable advancement, and you return to old procedures are terrible and unfulfilling. In any case, such as gaining "an inappropriate" course on the grand trekking trail, you'll see that outings into matured expending examples can be used as learning encounters. (Numerous climbers wouldn't ordinarily scold themselves to be uncertain of what direction to take; rather, they'd be grateful for the disclosures of character that a blocked course offered.) It's imperative that you help yourself out and welcome the preparation that turns out from experience. This procedure includes originating from a position of interest rather than a position of judgment, along these lines whatever you do; don't crush yourself up intellectually!

Intuitive Eating is very not equivalent to dieting. Dieters, for the most part, get disappointed on the off chance that they don't follow the dietary plan way decisively as endorsed. We've seen numerous a relentless dieters simply have an off-base change at one feast, be critical for that error, and "blow" the dietary plan for that day time or end of the week or in reality longer! Recall that the outing to Intuitive Eating is typically a procedure, loaded up with good and bad times, un-like dieting where in actuality the regular desire is unquestionably direct advancement (losing a specific measure of abundance weight in a specific time span).

The road to Intuitive Eating is like obtaining a long haul common store. Over the long haul, you will see an arrival on speculation, paying little mind to the everyday vacillations of the money markets. It is customary and anticipated. How amusing that individuals have been prepared that, in financial matters, the everyday changes in the cash markets are typical, and once in a while is there a moment get-rich fix, yet, in the multibillion-dollar, a year pounds misfortune business, "get slender quick" might be the main target for accomplishment. We are contributed, rather, in helping you give harmony to your expending presence and self-perception. In connection to this objective, remember Webster's portrayal of procedure: "a continuous advancement including numerous alterations" and "a particular way to deal with accomplishing something, including various advances or activities by and large."

Much like any procedure, it's essential that you remain centred in, and develop from the numerous experiences you will experience. Assuming, in any case, you focus on the result (which for some, people is fat or the number of pounds lost), it could make you experience overpowered and debilitated, and wrap up disrupting the strategy. Rather, if your air conditioning information little changes in transit and worth the preparation encounters (that may in some cases be disappointing), it can assist you with adhering to the Intuitive Eating course and push ahead. When you truly become an Intuitive Eater, you will consistently check out your inward insight, and you may feel better on a basic level, body, and soul.

Now, we feel it is important to explain the issue of the mission for weight reduction. For a few, the body will return to its normal abundance weight level, which might be not exactly your present pounds and remain there. To watch if this relates to you, ask yourself the following inquiries: Perhaps you have routinely destroyed from agreeable totality level? Perform you routinely gorge when you're getting arranged for the following diet (understanding that there will turn into a ton of foods you won't be allowed to eat on the dietary plan)? Perform your gorge as an adapting framework in troublesome events or to fill period when you're exhausted? Maybe you have been impervious to work out?

Do you only exercise in the event that you are dieting? Do you skip foods or hold back to eat until you're insatiably hungry, possibly to find that you indulge when you at long last expend? Do you are feeling remorseful; either when you indulge or when you take in all that you call a "poor food," which results in all the more overeating? If you addressed "yes" for a few of the vast majority of these inquiries, after that all things considered, your present weight might be more prominent than the weight the body is intended to keep up. Furthermore, it is likely you will have the option to return to your common, sound weight, because of this procedure. Be that as it may, recall, weight decrease should be put on the storage compartment burner. In the event that you focus on weight reduction, it'll meddle with your ability to settle on decisions predicated on your intuitive signs.

When you've surrendered the pointlessness of dieting perpetually, you'll wind up eating far fewer suppers with a craving to see customary movement in your day by day life. You'll find that the body feels so far superior when your midsection isn't stuffed, at whatever point your muscle tissue is conditioned, just as your heart is coordinate. You will likewise find that as your contemplations about your eating and body begin to transform, you will encounter an all the more loosening up feeling, rather than the incessant foundation stress that weaving machines each supper decision. Nonetheless, if you keep on focusing on weight decrease as the objective, you'll get tangled up in the matured diet-attitude figuring, which won't serve you.

Throughout the years, we've seen our people continue through a five-organize movement in figuring out how to be an Intuitive Eater. The following segment can assist you with getting an idea of what things to expect inside your very own adventure.

STAGE ONE: READINESS-HITTING DIET PLAN BOTTOM
This is the place numerous individuals start. You are agonizingly conscious that each attempt to get in shape is made in "falling flat." You are wary of esteeming every day predicated on whether the level is as a rule up or down a pound or two (or on the off chance that you indulged your prior day). You envision and stress over dinners constantly. You talk the prohibitive food visit "Just in the event that I didn't have to watch my overabundance weight, I could expend that," or "I encountered two treats I truly was awful today."

As of now, your weight might be higher than any time in recent memory, or, without significantly over-weight, you lose and increase five or ten pounds to such an extent and rapidly as you wash your garments in addition to they get filthy again! You have lost contact with organic food longings and satiety signals.

You have overlooked all that you truly prefer to expend and rather eat all that you figure you "should" eat. Your association with dinners has built up a poor tone, and you fear to eat the foods you like since you're apprehensive it'll be difficult to stop. At the point when you yield to the enticement of illegal foods, it's normal to indulge them, since you are feeling remorseful. However, you earnestly pledge you won't ever eat them again.

It's not bizarre to get that you take into comfort, occupy, or even numb yourself from your very own emotions. On the off chance that that is the situation, you will feel that an incredible evaluation offers been blurred by obsession thinking about suppers and by careless expending.

The self-perception is negative-you don't simply like the manner in which you show up and feel inside your body, and confidence is reduced. You have found from your experience that dieting won't work-you have arrived in a desperate predicament and experience stuck, debilitated, and disheartened.

This stage proceeds until you select that you will be troubled eating and living along these lines you will be prepared to accomplish something positive about it. Your first contemplations may veer toward finding another diet to determine your issues. Yet, very quickly, you comprehend that you can't do that one until kingdom come. On the off chance that that is the place you find yourself, you at that point are set up for the method that will empower you to get back again to eating intuitively.

STAGE TWO: EXPLORATION-CONSCIOUS LEARNING AND QUEST FOR PLEASURE

That is a phase of investigation and disclosure. You will continue through a phase of hyper consciousness to incredibly help reacquaint yourself together with your intuitive signs: hunger, season inclinations, and satiety.

This stage resembles figuring out how precisely to drive a vehicle. For the beginner driver, simply getting the vehicle out from the garage requires a lot of conscious deduction, loaded up with a psychological agenda: Place the principle component in the start, make certain the contraption is in diversion zone or impartial, start the motor, check the rearview reflect, remove the hand brake, and so forth. This hyper consciousness is basic to secure every one of the means required simply to acquire that vehicle into Drive! In a similar inclination, you will focus in on subtleties of eating which have advanced without such centred reasoning. (In any case, this is basic to recover the Intuitive Eater in you.)

It might seem clumsy and awkward, fanatical even. In any case, hyper consciousness varies than over the top considering. Over the top reasoning is generally unavoidable and is viewed as stress. It fills your brain during most of the day and prevents you from considering much else. Hyperconsciousness is increasingly specific. It zooms in the event that you have thought about food, yet leaves totally when the eating experience is finished. What's more, like the means required stresses become autopilot for the accomplished driver, Intuitive Eating will eventually get experienced without this fundamental ungainliness.

You may accept that you are in a hyperconscious state more often than not during this stage. This may feel awkward at first just as maybe even abnormal. Keep in mind, a ton of your prior eating was either primarily thoughtless or diet plan coordinated. In this stage, you'll begin to make harmony with food giving yourself unqualified consent to expend. This part may feel frightening, and you may choose to move gradually (inside your solace level). Become acquainted with to wipe out blame incited eating and begin to find the requirement for the fulfilment component with food. The significantly progressively cheerful you are while expending, the substantially less you see food on the off chance that you are not hungry you won't wind up being lurking here and there.

You will explore different avenues regarding foods that you probably won't have eaten for quite a while. This comprises of sifting through your exact food needs and needs. You may even find that you don't simply like the kind of a couple of the foods you've been longing for! (Remember those long stretches of dieting, or eating all that you "should" simply serve to disengage you from your own inner eating travel and genuine food decisions.) Become acquainted with to respect your food yearnings and perceive the body markers that show the innumerable degrees of appetite. Become acquainted with, to separate these organic pointers from the enthusiastic markers that may likewise trigger eating. In this stage, you may find that you will eat bigger degrees of foods than the body needs. It will be difficult to regard your totality as of now since you will require time to try out the amount it requires to satisfy a denied sense of taste. What's more, it requires some serious energy that you ought to create trust with suppers again and comprehend that it's really okay to expend. By what means will you respect completion, on the off chance that you are not absolutely sure it's okay to eat the specific food, or if you fear it won't become there tomorrow?

In the event that you have recently been putting on overabundance weight, weight gain typically stops or is restricted to just a couple of pounds. At the point when you have been utilizing suppers inwardly, you may find that you will begin to feel your emotions and may encounter uneasiness, pity, or really sadness on occasion. Most of your eating could be foods that are heavier in fat and sugar than you've been familiar with in spite of the fact that you may have been eating huge degrees of these food types furtively or with blame. How you eat in this stage will never be the example that you'll set up or requirement for a lifetime. You will see that your nourishing soundness is for the most part helter-skelter and you probably won't feel physically alongside focuses during this time. That is all standard and anticipated. You have to let yourself continue through this phase for such a long time as you need. Keep in mind, and you are creating for quite a while of hardship, troublesome self-talk, and blame. You are re-building positive food experiences, much the same as a strand of pearls. Every feast experience, similar to each pearl, may seem immaterial, however, by and large, they change lives.

STAGE THREE: CRYSTALLIZATION
In this stage, you will experience the primary renewals of the Intuitive Eating style which has consistently been a piece of you, yet was covered underneath the flotsam and jetsam of dieting. At the point when you enter this stage, a great deal of the investigation work from the earlier stage begins to solidify and feels as if strong conducts change. Your thoughts regarding food are not any more over the top. You barely need to stay aware of the hyperconsciousness about eating that was initially required. Thusly, your eating choices don't require very as particularly coordinated accepted. Rather, you find that your food choices and reactions to natural pointers are principally intuitive.

You have a bigger feeling of trust-both in your to pick what you really need to eat and in the undeniable reality that your natural signs are depend-capable. You are advantageous with your food choices and will start to see expanded satisfaction at your suppers.

Now, you respect your appetite most of the time and it's less difficult to perceive what you feel simply like eating in the event that you are hungry. You keep on creating harmony with food.

What feels new in this stage is that it's more straightforward to require some investment out in the midst of your food to intentionally check exactly how a lot of your paunch is topping off. It is conceivable to watch your completion and regard the presence of that sign, regardless of whether you find that you as often as possible eat past the totality tag. Precisely like when a toxophilite requires focus on a crisp objective, it frequently requires catching numerous bolts before figuring out how precisely to come to the bull's-eye. You may at present be picking recently prohibited foods most of the time, yet you will find that you don't require as a lot of them to satisfy you.

On the off chance that you've been a genuinely signaled eater, you'll become very skilled at isolating natural yearning markers from passionate appetite. Because of this lucidity, more than not frequently, you'll be encountering your feelings and discovering techniques to com-stronghold and occupy yourself without the use of food.

Be certain you put weight decrease on the storage compartment burner. Much more significant than abundance weight reduction, is the inclination of well-turning out to be and strengthening that become-gins to happen. You won't any longer feel vulnerable and miserable. You will begin to regard your body and get that in case you're over your regular weight, it's because of the dieting attitude, rather than absence of resolve.

STAGE 4: THE INTUITIVE EATER AWAKENS
By enough time you arrive at this stage, all the work you have just been doing comes full circle in an agreeable, free-streaming eating style. You consistently pick what you truly need to eat when you are ravenous. Since you comprehend that you can have altogether more suppers, based on your personal preference, when you are starving, it's anything but difficult to stop eating when you are feeling serenely full.

You may begin to find that you pick more advantageous foods, not on the grounds that you envision you should, but since you are feeling better physically when you take along these lines.

The pressing need to demonstrate to yourself that you could have recently prohibited foods could have reduced. You truly know and trust these foods will be there, and on the off chance that you need to eat them truly, you can-in this manner they drop their charming quality. Chocolate starts to shield myself against a similar mental implication as a peach. You won't any more drawn out need to test yourself, just as your hardship reaction with suppers will be no more.

At the point when you do choose the foods you used to limit, you'll get extraordinary delight, and feel content with a particularly littler amount than beforehand, and without blame. (At the point when you are feeling regretful eating a suppers, it removes a great deal of the happiness from eating.)

In the event that managing your emotions have been hard for you, you'll be less reluctant to see them, and be increasingly capable at plunking down with them. Finding refreshing choices to occupy and comfort yourself when required can be normal for you.

Your food talk and self talk will be certain and non-basic. Your tranquility settlement with suppers is solidly settled, and you will have discharged any contention or remaining blame about dinner's decisions you have hauled around.

You have quit being furious together with your body and making ill bred input about it. You regard it and acknowledge there are a wide range of shapes and sizes on the planet. At this genuine point, and if it's intended to be, the body will be coming to moving toward its natural weight.

STAGE FIVE: THE ULTIMATE STAGE-TREASURE THE PLEASURE
Right now your Intuitive Eater has been guaranteed. You will confide in your body's intuitive capacities it will be easy to respect your yearning and regard totality. At long last, you will encounter no blame about your feast decisions or amounts. Since you like your sentimental relationship to dinners and fortune the fulfillment that eating currently offers you, you will dispose of unacceptable eating conditions and unappealing foods.

You should encounter benefiting from in the most ideal of conditions as opposed to corrupt it with enthusiastic misery. You will encounter an internal conviction to quit utilizing food to deal with enthusiastic circumstances, if that is your propensity. At the point when sentiments become too astounding, you will see that you'll much rather adapt to your feelings or occupy yourself at times from their site with anything separated from food.

Since your eating style has become a wellspring of joy rather than a suffering, you will encounter sustenance and development in various manners.

The duty of activity will be evacuated, and practicing will begin to look luring to you. Exercise won't be used as a driving strain to catch fire more calories; rather, you feel com-mitted to exercise with an end goal to feel much improved, and intellectually physically. In like manner, food won't be another instrument to make you feel terrible about how you eat; rather, it transforms into an approach to feeling as in reality great and solid as could be expected under the circumstances.

At the point when you arrive at a definitive stage, your bodyweight will sink into what's normal for you-a spot that is agreeable and befitting your height and body outline. In the event that your bodyweight was at that point ordinary, you will find that you'll keep up it without exertion and you will be freed of the mental good and bad times that go with the confinement/overeating cycles.

Finally, you will encounter enabled and shielded from outside powers telling you what and exactly the amount to eat, and how the body should look. You will feel clear of the duty of dieting. What's more, you'll be an Intuitive Eater again.

THAT YOU CAN DO IT!
These stages and the progressions that happen with your eating and considerations may seem outlandish. Or on the other hand, it may show up excessively startling. For instance, the very idea of giving yourself unrestricted authorization to eat may seem unnerving and you may expect that you'll never stop eating or

putting on abundance weight. The remainder of the distribution clarifies in extraordinary fine detail how precisely to execute every rule, why it truly is required, and the explanation behind it. Also, you will figure out how extra interminable dieters became Intuitive Eaters and how it changed their lives. By enough time you wrap up this book, you will unquestionably realize that you also may turn into an Intuitive Eater, and forestall the franticness of dieting.

Conclusion

Thank you for reading this book!

Now you have all the instructions to perform Atkins Diet in the best possible way!

CPSIA information can be obtained
at www.ICGtesting.com
Printed in the USA
BVHW041324201120
593807BV00005B/93

9 781801 201094